Dear Liz

Thank you for
doing what you do.

Love Kate.

I WISH MY DOCTOR HAD TOLD ME THIS

I WISH MY DOCTOR HAD TOLD ME THIS

There is more to our healing than medication

KATE CHAYTOR-NORRIS

First published in Great Britain in 2020 by Tigga Publishing

Illustrations by Nor Brown

Edited, designed and produced by Tandem Publishing
http://tandempublishing.yolasite.com

ISBN: 978-1-5272-6061-0

10 9 8 7 6 5 4 3 2 1

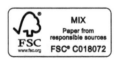

A CIP catalogue record for this book is available from the British Library.

Printed and bound in Great Britain by CPICPI Group (UK) Ltd, Croydon CR0 4YY.

For my family
In huge gratitude.

To my husband Trevor
For his inordinate patience and support when I
introduce another eccentric element into my life or
keep moving the goalposts and for all of those times
when I say 'I'm just off to do another course!'

To G
For embracing my world and encouraging and
helping me to write this book.

To Pose
A most courageous warrior and my greatest teacher.

To Harry
For giving the best hugs in the whole world, having
the modus operandi 'Stressing doesn't help' and
writing beautiful songs that make me cry.

Contents

'No matter how much it gets abused, the body can restore balance. The first rule is to stop interfering with nature.'

— Deepak Chopra

INTRODUCTION

My reasons for writing this book arose from a passion for the prevention of disease. So much better to deal with it *before* it develops, rather than trying to find a cure once it has taken root. Time and time again I sit with a client and, when I explain what is going on in their bodies, they ask me, 'Why didn't my doctor / specialist tell me this … it makes so much sense?' Working out the underlying causes of disease is key, and by addressing those causes we can help the body regain balance. I started to run workshops to spread the word, but this was a drop-in-the-ocean approach. So here is my next endeavour, a book explaining those underlying causes, and a presentation of the strategies that my clients and I over time have found to be most effective.

The crux of the problem lies in the fact that our bodies have not yet adapted to deal with 21st-century living. We are inextricably linked to our environment, and in order to thrive we need to improve our adaptation. This is a challenging proposition when you look at the speed of change in our environment. The developments in the last fifty years alone are breathtaking, but not always for the good. Our bodies are seeking a more hospitable habitat, one in which we can be more at ease in this accelerated world.

Evolution is a glacially slow and steady process; in order for our bodies really to cope in today's world, we would all need massive adrenal glands to handle the stress, giant livers to deal with the number of toxins and enormous pancreases for insulin production to cope with the levels of sugar and refined carbohydrates. The speed at which our environment and society have changed has simply left us behind. Our bodies speak a language: they are constantly giving us feedback about what is beneficial or not. The symptoms that they produce are there to tell us that our systems are out of balance ... but because we are too busy and hectic we don't take the time to listen.

With rates of chronic disease soaring, it is important that we take a long hard look at the environment we live in. Taking medicine alone will not change the environment and bring back balance; pills are a sticking-plaster approach to healing, suppressing symptoms instead of dealing with underlying causes. Pharmaceutical companies pour millions of pounds into researching the next big drug that will make them a fortune, so there is huge pressure to prescribe in order to recoup expenses and of course make profits. It is up to us to become a little more discerning about what we put into our bodies and take responsibility for changing the environmental factors that are pushing us out of kilter. The aim is to create a nutritious and nurturing habitat for our bodies and minds to thrive. As I write these lines in early spring 2020 the whole world is in the grip of a health crisis – Covid-19. If there was ever a time where we need to be putting our health and immunity at the forefront, this is it. A time for us to take responsibility for our own health and that of our community.

As a Nutritional Therapist, my focus is very much on nourishing food, but diet change is not always the magic bullet. If people are experiencing chronic disease, rarely is it only one factor causing the symptoms. This is why a functional medicine approach, which looks at the body as a whole and ascertains the underlying imbalances, has so much more success in healing than medication.

Nutritional suggestions will always be my primary focus with a client; however, experience has taught me that the mind and soul also need to be nourished. In fact I would go as far as to say that chronic disease is a manifestation of what is occurring on an emotional level; the emotional baggage we carry around dictates the lens through which we perceive everything – this can profoundly impact the way we live our lives and how our bodies function.

In the words of Carl Jung: 'When an inner situation is not made conscious, it happens outside, as fate…'

This discovery of the huge emotional component of disease led me to train in all sorts of different therapies, so I can look at clients from all sorts of different angles. My methods, as well as nutrition, include health kinesiology which incorporates some Chinese Medicine principles, face reading, which can give me clues about a person's emotional journey as well as organs that may be out of balance, and also PSYCH-K® training to help the body release trapped emotions.

On my journey as a therapist I have made numerous discoveries about myself, not all of them comfortable, and I will share those with you in the hope that they may help you realise you are not alone. I hope that I have managed to not sound too preachy – please forgive me if I have. Keep in mind that even though I am fully aware of the benefits that can be gained through adhering to my own advice, it doesn't mean that I always manage to achieve it. I see myself as a constant work in progress, chipping away at the coal-face. But when I do get it right the results are well worth it.

I hope you will find this book useful. In dealing with many of the subjects here, what you will read is my honest opinion, and some of the conclusions have not necessarily been scientifically proven, but proof, as you will read later, is a bit of a slippery subject. I have divided up the important factors that need attention into the 5 Ss – Stress, Sugar, Sludge (toxins), Sleep and Spirit. My aim is to offer you a few tools that may help you achieve a healthy, thriving body and mind. Admittedly we all start from varying degrees of health and vitality. Our experiences, in particular during childhood, plus the inherited baggage of our parents and past generations, all play a part in shaping us. Then there is the genetic component, about which we have all been misled. Our genetic expression depends upon the environment that our genes are exposed to – 'Genes load the gun but the environment pulls the trigger' sums up the situation perfectly.

Despite differing life experiences and genetics, it is possible for each and every one of us to create the optimal internal and external environments to suit our individual bodies. The only hitch is that it does take some homework. I am blessed and forever grateful that my clients are prepared to take on the challenge to heal their bodies and regain energy, vitality and joyous wellbeing. That happy state is one that should be – and is – available to us all.

— Kate Chaytor-Norris
Spring 2020

1

EVOLUTION

(OR LACK OF IT)

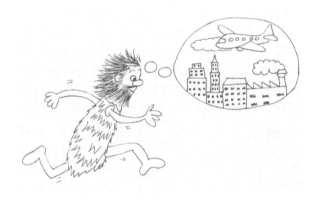

The evolution of our bodies is just not happening fast enough. The speed at which society has developed in the last 50 years is quite mind-boggling, expecially when we compare the pace of development since man first arrived on this planet approximately 900,000 years ago. Back then, humans lived as hunter-gatherers, foraging for food, experiencing extremes of temperature, facing daily challenges to the immune system. They lived in close communities[1] (essential for survival) where everyone worked together for a common cause and there was time to rest and rebalance the body. On a psychological level it is a world that 'we subconsciously still inhabit' (Yuval Noah Harari *Sapiens*)[2] but the problem is that we are being bombarded with so much more, work strain, money worries, toxins and societal pressures. All of these are tipping the body over the edge to where it has to produce symptoms, many of which are expressed by imbalances in our mental wellbeing.[3] The physical and mental health of the modern world is in crisis, which is not surprising when you compare our present world to the one from which we have descended.

OUR ANCIENT ANCESTORS ACTUALLY HAD IT
BETTER (MOSTLY...)

Let's rewind to when we were living in caves: generally, life was simple. We may have had our stress response triggered perhaps once a day at the very most, hunting for food or fighting off a sabre-toothed tiger / woolly mammoth, all of which were pretty extreme events. However, there was always an element of downtime: once the food and shelter question had been dealt with, then it was time for rest, relaxation and socialising. This type of 'leisure time' was very different to now. It might have been staring into the fire, playing with some sticks or stones, rolling around on the cave floor with the children, discussing the latest hunting adventure or admiring the sunset – by modern standards possibly rather boring. These simple pastimes would generally have been carried out with complete focus, as there wasn't that incessant bombardment of outside data streaming in. This more focused and mindful existence would have allowed the body to maintain homeostasis – a state of equilibrium when heart rates, blood pressure and stress hormone levels would have all come back into balance, allowing the body to regenerate and repair.

This simple unadulterated spare time would also have allowed proper connection with other humans – *full* attention given to another person, with no distraction from mobiles / TV / radio / computers etc. When we fully attend to someone else, face to face, the communication is so much more profound and accurate, all nuances of facial expression and body language coming into play. There is far less room for misinterpretation, no opportunity for the miscommunications that can occur with electronic messages, leading to so much conflict and unhappiness.

Human beings are wired for connection and without that connection we do not thrive. Lord Winston, who has produced documentaries like *Child of our Time*, stated in a paper, 'The importance of early bonding on the long-term mental health and resilience of children', 'There is increasing evidence from the fields of development psychology, neurobiology and animal epigenetic studies that neglect, parental inconsistency and a lack of love can lead to long-term mental health problems as well as to reduced overall potential and happiness.'[4]

CONNECTION WITH NATURE

The hunter-gatherer existence would have provided ample contact with mother nature – no rubber / plastic-soled shoes, concrete foundations, tarmacked areas and general indoor existence. There is much scientific evidence to show that our bodies are energetically linked with mother earth, our body's bio-rhythms affected by tides, seasons, phases of the moon, and the free source of antioxidants provided by her. This is a vital part of our long-term wellbeing and something that for most of us has been lost. I will look at this further in the SPIRIT Chapter.

THE PERILS OF 'MAN-MADE'

In the past there was a distinct lack of laboratories to create toxic chemicals. With scientific advances, we have created weird and wonderful combinations of elements in a bid to make our lives 'easier'. Now our environment is loaded with these substances, most of which have a detrimental effect upon our systems. We have created chemical combinations that are just not recognised by the human body – toxins: therefore, the body feels constantly under attack and has to treat them as the enemy. Our liver, the main organ in charge of detoxing most 'foreign' or excess substances, is getting seriously overloaded.

OUR ANCESTORS DIDN'T SIT

The life of a hunter-gatherer was hugely physical in comparison to current modern standards; anywhere you needed to be or anything that you needed to acquire involved movement and expending energy. If they did rest, it would not involve lounging in a chair, but probably squatting, which stretches the lower back muscles, increases the mobility of our hips and does not compress the spine. Our bodies are built for movement. In an attempt to reduce the amount of time that I sit in front of my computer, I have purchased a standing-up desk. It took a little bit of time to get used to, and my legs ached like mad to start off with, but eventually my body adjusted. It also made me much more aware of my posture: if I don't stand properly my body will really start to shout at me. I have to admit here, with regard to taking exercise, I am not necessarily an advocate of pounding on the treadmill in the gym, in fact I don't do running. I envy those people that can go off for a run, get in the zone and come back feeling fantastic … but that just is not me. If we look at our ancestors, it is unlikely that they would have run for miles – short sharp bursts to fight or run away (much more in line with HIIT – High Intensity Interval Training) but the rest would have been walking, possibly very long distances, and general movement – no hours sat at a desk or watching just another episode.

The most important thing is *to keep moving*; I am sure

that you have heard the phrase 'Sitting is the new smoking', coined by Dr James Levine – well this is why. Studies have shown that those who spend the majority of their day sitting have an increased risk for cancer, heart disease, obesity, Type 2 diabetes, cognitive decline and depression. One of the main problems with being sedentary is that it affects the flow of cerebrospinal fluid (CSF). CSF cushions the brain, but it is also vital for delivering nutrients and taking away waste products. An undernourished and dirty brain is not going to function properly and this will impact the entire body. There is also the effect of not burning the calories that we should, hence the higher risk for obesity, diabetes, cancer and heart disease. I will expand on these health issues and their underlying causes later. Furthermore, a sedentary body means that lymph flow is hampered: this is a system that helps to clean the blood and fight infection and it relies upon muscle contraction for proper functioning.

Doctors should be prescribing more activity – any which way we can get our bodies moving will help. This can be very challenging when you have a desk job, and some forward-thinking companies are starting to invest in standing / treadmill desks, but just getting up from your desk every 30 minutes for a stretch and a quick walk about can improve the situation. I know of one practitioner who has a trampette in her office – she schedules 5 minutes between appointments so she can spend 3 minutes bouncing.

HUNTER-GATHERER CUISINE

The hunter-gatherer diet was generally far superior to ours – none of the food would have been fast-tracked and refined, it would have been chemical-free, slow grown, pasture-fed, antibiotic-free woolly mammoth or fish with a large proportion of plant matter. The animals would have grazed on a huge variety of vegetation, vegetation that itself would have grown in nutrient-rich soil where climate and agriculture would not have been contributing to its deficiencies.

These hunter-gatherers would have eaten a wide variety of foods and they would also have eaten seasonally, so the immune system would not have been exposed to the same foods day after day.

The fat content was also much higher – when an animal was killed and eaten, every bit of the fat was consumed, as this provided exceptional fuel – 1gm of fat will provide 9 calories of energy, whereas 1gm of carbohydrate will provide 4 calories of energy. I can hear the fat-phobic community getting ansty here, and I will explain later that fat is GOOD for us, not the demon that causes heart disease (the UK's largest killer). Another point I would also like to make, whilst on the subject of calories, is that I do not advocate calorie counting – a boring and tedious pastime, and more importantly much misinformation abounds about calorie intake. See FOOD Chapter. Weight gain does not necessarily depend on the amount of calories consumed – it makes a huge difference *which* type of foods those calories come from.

Possible hunter-gatherer food diary
Although there is much debate about the exact components of a hunter-gatherer diet, the very earliest evidence of farming is 23,000 years ago[5] so we can be sure that their diet was much less carbohydrate-based. Weapons to kill larger prey were not developed until 500,000 years ago so the initial hunter-gatherers would have only consumed smaller prey unless there was a large beast that had died of natural causes.[6] After this date it is likely that animal protein consumption would have increased. The incorporation of larger amounts of animal protein was essential for the evolution of the larger human brain.[7]

It is likely that they would have eaten once a day if lucky – 3 meals a day is merely a social construct.

- One meal of some sort of animal, if they had managed to catch something, otherwise it would have been foraged food, lots of plant matter, roots, nuts, seeds. There is likely to have been a much greater variety of plant matter consumed – they would have eaten whatever was available, not their favourite item from a supermarket shelf.
- Fruit if it was in season.
- Water

Typical 21ˢᵗ-century food diary
- Breakfast – cereal / 'healthy' muesli (many mueslis are packed with sugar); Toast with jam / marmalade / chocolate spread with nuts etc; Coffee / tea
- Lunch – sandwich possibly containing a little salad, crisps, chocolate bar, fizzy drink
- Supper – pasta, rice or potatoes with processed meat / fish and perhaps a few vegetables – glass or two of wine / beer / spirits
- Some kind of sugar to assuage that desire for 'a little something sweet'.

I may be doing you a disservice here, but I am going off an average of what my clients are eating when they arrive at my door.

It is likely that the hunter-gatherers eating once a day would have taken time over their meals, giving themselves the opportunity to digest their food, not rushing off to the next appointment or meeting. Due to the higher fat and unrefined sugars in the diet, their blood sugar control will have been excellent, allowing them to fast for long periods without starting to feel floppy, dizzy, shaky and brain foggy. See section on SUGAR for more on this and the benefits of intermittent fasting.

The more you can reduce your carbs (bread, pasta, potatoes, rice, biscuits, cakes) and sugar intake the better. I know it sounds scary and, for some, almost impossible when you look at how carbohydrate-based our diets have become, but if you put your mind to it anything is possible – see carb alternatives in FOOD Chapter. The most important thing from my experience is that initially you do not allow yourself to get too hungry – that is when the biscuit tin will start calling and your willpower dial will be turned to zero. Once your blood sugar levels start to balance, I am a fan of intermittent fasting. One thing that I have got up my sleeve that may help you to feel more satisfied (and not feel the need to raid the sweetie jar) with your low-carbohydrate meal is that you can increase the fat. It is not helpful, however, to increase the fat and still eat the carbs / sugar – that would be having your cake and eating it, so to speak. We have been brainwashed that fat causes heart disease and this is one of the reasons why we have such obesity problems. The low-fat industry is huge and powerful with, quite understandably, a mission to make foods that taste good. The problem with removing fat from food is that it loses its flavour, so the only option is to add sugar, salt, MSG etc – a disaster for those wanting to lose weight. Clients, especially my weight-loss clients, are often shocked and sometimes a little suspicious when I ask them to stop buying any low-fat products and go for the full-fat version.

The misinformation about fat started in the 1950s when a man named Dr Ancel Keys set about proving that consumption of saturated fat was linked to cardiovascular disease. He travelled around the world gathering data from 22 countries. He then returned back home, cherry-picked statistics from a few of those countries, neglecting for example to use the data from the Eskimos, who had a very high-fat diet (all that whale and seal blubber) and low levels of cardiovascular disease. This very unfortunate manipulation of data started the low-fat ball rolling. Any way that manufacturers could remove fat from the diet could only be a good thing, right? Roll in the low-fat industry and inventions like margarine (polyunsaturated fat), which is really a first cousin of plastic. Or a more ludicrous recent idea of the low-fat industry, selling egg whites only! More recent studies have shown that there is no correlation between saturated fat consumption and heart disease.[8] We will delve into the causes of cardiovascular disease in a later chapter.

If you are still suspicious about my advocating fat as a better fuel see the FOOD Chapter for a more detailed look. You can also look at *Fat for Fuel* by Dr Joseph Mercola.

***

At one of the very first lectures when I started training as a Nutritional Therapist, the lecturer started with 'Hello my name is Patrick and I am 45; if I told you I was still breastfeeding you would think me a little strange.' Well, that certainly got our attention. The last element of the hunter-gatherer diet worth noting is a lack of dairy consumption. Our lecturer then went on to explain the problems with our modern ways. No other animal continues to consume milk into adulthood – yet that is exactly what humans do. Milk is for babies and growing children – it contains growth hormones, which can promote the growth of cancer cells (we all have cancerous cells in our body all the time; it is up to a healthy immune system to seek out and destroy them). Milk also contains oestrogen: some has higher levels than others, as some dairy cows are treated with oestrogen-like hormones to boost milk supplies. In 2000, Professor Jane Plant was one of the first people to raise this issue, when dealing with cancer herself she researched the link between dairy consumption and breast cancer. She found that the rates of breast cancer in countries where they do not consume dairy, like China, were 1 in 100,000, when ours in the West was 1 in 10 (it is now 1 in 8). She also found that the Chinese women, if they moved to the West and adopted a Western diet, which included dairy, increased their risk to the same level as ours, so it is not a genetic issue. I am not necessarily saying that we should never consume dairy but perhaps we should be watchful of how much we are ingesting. It is very easy for levels to mount up: milk on cereal or yoghurt at breakfast, cheese sandwich or cheesy / sour-cream baked potato for lunch, cheese and biscuits, cheesy sauces, ice cream / yoghurt for supper. We all tend to be creatures of habit, so eat similar things every day. You may find that your diet is quite dairy-heavy.

One last thing to say about dairy – there are a growing number of people who are intolerant to dairy. In my experience some of those that can't digest it are fine when they start consuming raw milk. This is for two reasons: firstly, raw milk is not pasteurised (this is a heat treatment that kills the bacteria; this process also kills all the enzymes that would help us to digest the milk). Some people have more lactase and protease enzymes naturally occurring in their systems than others, the ones who don't have to rely on the enzymes contained in the milk to help them break down the lactase sugar and the milk protein. Secondly, raw milk is not homogenised (this is a mechanical process where the fat globules are broken down to smaller droplets so that the milk does not separate out into the cream on the top and the milk underneath). I remember as a small child, when we had a dairy farm, the daily ritual of collecting the milk from the farm, putting it in a large bowl and waiting for the cream to rise to the top then skimming it off. There were very few dairy allergies / intolerances in those days compared to now. The problem with homogenisation of the fat in milk is that the human body does not recognise this alien structure of fat and treats it as an invader. Homogenised milk also releases an enzyme, xanthine oxidase, into the body; in the 1960s Kurt Oster discovered that there was a link between this enzyme and higher rates of cardiovascular disease.[9]

HUNTER-GATHERER CURES

Thanks to pioneering DNA work we now have more information about the health of the ancient hunter-gatherers. Data shows that they did not die of chronic diseases like diabetes and heart disease, it was more likely to be infection, starvation and accidents. I hear the argument that hunter-gatherers did not live long enough to develop chronic disease (usually about 30–35 years old) but chronic disease is starting to appear in our modern population well before the age of 30–35.[10] [11]

It is difficult to ascertain what the hunter-gatherers used for medicine, as there was nothing written down to pass on to future generations. One of the first medical documents is the Ebers Papyrus, an Egyptian medical document of herbal knowledge dating to c.1550 BC, which showed the use of dates, honey, acacia and elderberry. Half an onion and the froth of beer was considered 'a delightful remedy against death'.

Over time, there have been many effective plant-based remedies used that work with the body, supporting it in its bid to maintain balance. Sadly, today we have got to a stage where mostly the 'remedies' that people are taking are chemically manufactured so that they can be patented. The statistics on Adverse Drug Reactions (ADRs) are eye-popping. Research shows that ADRs could be contributing to up to 22,303 deaths a year in the UK. Jeremy Hunt, the Health and Social Care Secretary at the time of writing, has berated the NHS for 'totally preventable' mistakes that are causing 'appalling levels' of harm. I had a client that came to me the other day who was on 12 different medications, 3 of which should not have been prescribed together, but we have become such a pill-popping culture this is accepted as the norm. The tragedy is that when patients go to the doctor, they are not informed that there is another way if they want to take their health into their own hands.

Our 21ˢᵗ-century bodies are really up against it – living in a world where our diet is so alien compared to what would naturally keep it healthy and thriving, our exposure to new toxins is overwhelming, we have a health system that does not have the ability to heal the body and our lifestyles are just too fast and packed for any sort of balance to be maintained.

Over the next few chapters I will look more closely at the real issues in our environment that drive the mechanisms of chronic diseases, and what we can do about them to help protect our bodies against an environment that is really not fit for human consumption.

2

ALL CHRONIC DISEASE IS PREVENTABLE

Chronic diseases don't happen overnight. Most of them have been brewing in the system for decades: it starts with cell damage which grows into tissue damage, which then starts to affect the function of an organ … and only then do we start to get symptoms. The body is a most miraculous machine that works so hard to keep everything balanced but eventually it has to send you a message in the form of symptoms to tell you that all is not well.

Many of us choose to ignore those niggly symptoms – don't make a fuss, don't be so self-focused, just live with it, it's not that bad. So, the body has to shout louder, giving you symptoms that are less easy to ignore. It is really important that we take note and try to understand what the body is asking for. I can assure you high cholesterol is not a statin deficiency and anxiety is not a deficiency in anti-depressants or beta-blockers. Our bodies speak a language, it is imperative that we listen and work out what the problem is if we want to avoid long-term chronic disease. Below are some of the major diseases whose rates are rising at a frightening speed:

- CARDIOVASCULAR / HEART DISEASE
- RESPIRATORY DISEASES
- CANCER
- TYPE 2 DIABETES
- ALZHEIMER'S AND DEMENTIA
- AUTOIMMUNE DISEASE

Before we move on to talk about specific diseases it would be remiss of me to ignore the genetic question. Our genes are continuously interacting with our environment. The body is constantly trying to adapt to all the new aspects of the 21st century that are being thrown at it, this includes regular redesigning of our systems to enable the body to function optimally. Gene expression is something that is malleable because the environment can determine whether genes are switched on or off, this is the body 'adapting' and sometimes that adaptation produces symptoms. If we can improve the environmental load, we can reduce the negative expression of genes, even if you have been dealt rather a bum deal on the genetic front.

CARDIOVASCULAR / HEART DISEASE

This is the number 1 killer in the world. 7 million people in the UK are living with heart disease and today 420 people will lose their lives here to this preventable condition. The arteries, veins and capillaries that make up the cardiovascular system are responsible for delivering nutrients, oxygen and chemical messengers to all the cells in the body. If this system is malfunctioning then it will have a profound effect on every single part of the body.

I would like to start with, for most, the revolutionary idea that:

THE HEART IS NOT THE ONLY MECHANISM FOR GETTING BLOOD AROUND THE BODY

Our blood vessels placed end to end would stretch twice around the world – that is approximately 50,000 miles. Some of our capillaries are so tiny that the red blood cells have to change shape to squeeze through them. It is a physical impossibility that the heart's contraction is powerful enough to force a viscous fluid that distance with so much resistance. So how does blood travel around the body?

It has been observed that the blood, as it flows, goes at different speeds depending upon whether it is in the arteries, capillaries or veins – no surprise there, but what is surprising is that blood flow stops when it is in the capillaries (this is necessary for the exchange of oxygen and nutrients) but then it starts again and flows into the veins. Research into this phenomenon has ascertained that it is not the heart that is making the blood move: it is connected to the nature of water.

Dr Gerald Pollack, a leading research scientist in the field of physics, discovered that water has four states: not only can it be in the form of solid, liquid or gas, it can also exist in the form of structured water or gel phase. This form of water is the state of most of the water within our bodies, otherwise we would have a huge problem of leakage from cells.

Bear with me here: this is where we need to indulge in a bit of chemistry. If we look at the wall of a blood vessel we see that it is hydrophilic, which means water-loving. Any water-loving surface when it comes into contact with water creates a thin layer of this gel phase on its surface. The gel phase of water is negatively charged because it contains an excess of free electrons. So, imagine you have a tube with a thin layer of negatively charged gel phase water on its inside surface and then you have the blood flowing through (blood is 50% water). The water in the blood is positively charged with excess protons because the bulk of the negatively charged electrons are in the gel phase water. The positively-charged protons in the water of the blood repel each other and this creates the flow.

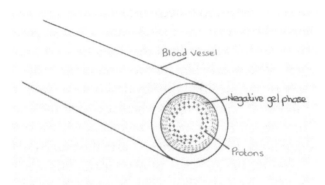

You may be thinking at this point, 'Why is she telling me this stuff? This is just a function happening in the body that I can't do anything about,' but that is the exciting bit; we can all help with this process. One vital factor for this whole system to work is the energy input, the energy that is required to maintain the gel phase of water by separating the electrons and protons to create the flow in the blood vessel. This energy comes from infra-red frequencies, e.g. sunlight or the electromagnetic field of the earth. This is one of the reasons why it is so fundamental to our health to get out into the sunshine – I know it is tricky if you live in the northern hemisphere, but you can always increase your contact with nature and mother earth. See SPIRIT Chapter. In his book *Human Heart, Cosmic Heart,* Thomas Cowan explores this fascinating phenomenon in depth.

The other system that is important to keep in balance, in order to ensure that our blood continues to flow freely through our blood vessels, is the autonomic nervous system. This nervous system has two parts, the Sympathetic – fight / flight nervous system – and the Parasympathetic – rest and digest nervous system. Those people who spend too much of their time in fight / flight mode due to chronic levels of stress run a much greater risk of a heart attack.

How does stress affect the cardiovascular system?
Major trauma can actually change the shape of your heart. The work of Sandeep Jauhar shows that in the first few weeks after a major shock or trauma, the heart becomes much more rounded; this is officially called Broken Heart Syndrome. It is thought that the very high levels of stress hormones actually prevent the heart from pumping properly and up to 20% of people with this syndrome can have a heart attack.

When we are in fight / flight mode, our body believes that it is in a life-threatening situation so very understandably it:

1. Increases the blood pressure to get the blood round faster so that the muscles have more nutrients and oxygen to be able to fight or flight. The problem with this is that increased pressure on the blood vessel walls means there is a greater likelihood of damage to the delicate lining of the blood vessel. Any damage to the blood vessel wall will produce inflammation, which is effectively the activation of the immune system, the body's first line of defence.

Inflammation is evident in all chronic disease
When we have an injury that requires acute inflammation (pain, redness, swelling, heat) this is a good thing – the body is telling us there is a problem and it is healing itself. We need to rest and take care of that part of the body. However, when that inflammation becomes chronic it then causes a myriad of problems.

So back to our blood vessel where the immune sysem has been activated. A message will then travel to the liver to ask for cholesterol to be sent, because cholesterol is the healing agent that will be used to patch up damage in any blood vessel wall (cholesterol has been given a very bad rap but I hope by the time you have finished this book you may view it more positively). A combination of immune cells and cholesterol builds on the inside of the blood vessel wall, in order to try and fix the situation – this is called atherosclerotic plaque. If the plaque builds too much in the blood vessels that feed the heart, it restricts blood flow and can lead to a lack of oxygen and nutrients getting through which then leads to a heart attack. This is the conventional view of how we have heart attacks; however, mother nature is one step ahead of us. Studies show that if there are blockages in blood vessels, the body will develop a network of other smaller blood vessels around it, to compensate for the lack of blood flow through the main artery: this is called anastomosis.

2. Stress thickens the blood[12] so we don't bleed to death if we get injured in our life-threatening situation. Thicker blood is more likely to clot and does not flow so freely. Fibrinogen, one of the major clotting factors, is considered an important risk factor for heart attacks, e.g. your levels of fibrinogen in a blood test are a very good indicator for your risk of having a heart attack.[13]

3. Stress increases the amount of sugar in the bloodstream to provide energy for the muscles to fight or run. This makes sense, but the downside is that it forces the heart to swap the fuel that it burns for muscle contraction. A healthy heart likes to use fatty acids and ketones as its fuel (ketones are water-soluble energy molecules that are made in the liver from stored fat), but with adrenalin in the system caused by stress which increases blood sugar levels, the heart cells are forced to use glucose as a fuel source. When we burn glucose, one of the metabolic products is lactic acid and if there is a steep rise in lactic acid the change in pH (acidity / alkalinity) can paralyse the heart cells, leading to a heart attack.

This stress response is inappropriately preparing us for that life-threatening situation, something that rarely happens in the 21st century. Our stress is more likely to be the ongoing

KATE CHAYTOR-NORRIS

chronic worry of modern life that is packed far too full, but the body can't tell the difference, so it reacts to keep us safe.

In addition to the above factors there is the effect of nutritional deficiencies or excesses on the cardiovascular system:

Lack of essential fats (oily fish and nuts and seeds) can mean that we are not eating natural anti-inflammatories. Essential fat also helps to keep our blood more runny so that it is less likely to clot.

Lack of magnesium – magnesium is a natural antihypertensive which as far back as the 1980s has been shown to reduce blood pressure.[14]

Lack of antioxidants (brightly coloured pigments in fruits and vegetables). Oxidation is part of the inflammatory process which drives cardiovascular disease. Cholesterol only becomes problematic when it is oxidised. Eating a diet rich in antioxidants can dampen down the damage that oxidation creates in the body.

Excess sugar – too much sugar in the bloodstream causes damage by sticking to things like the blood vessel walls: this promotes inflammation.

Niacin deficiency – niacin can help to increase your levels of HDL 'good' cholesterol. Niacin is vitamin B3, a totally natural nutrient but the pharmaceutical industry has managed to make a synthetic version so that it can be patented. If you do want to experiment with this natural supplement then I would advise that you get the NO FLUSH niacin. For some people, even at low doses, niacin can produce a full body flush, this is not harmful but can be a little alarming. A niacin flush is when all of the surface capillaries in the skin become engorged with blood – a bit like flushing through the pipes! During one of my detox sessions I decided to have an Epsom salts bath and take some niacin to produce this flush which can increase the detox. My husband walked in: 'Oh my

19

God, what's happened to you' was the comment, as I stood there, bright red from top to toe. I suggest that if you want to experiment with niacin that you do it under the supervision of a BANT-registered Nutritional Therapist who can guide you through the process.

Before we leave the heart and cardiovascular system, I want to mention that the heart is so much more than 'just a pump': it is a surveillance system for the body, sending a huge amount of information up to the brain about our environment. (See SPIRIT Chapter for more on this.)

RESPIRATORY DISEASES
20% of the UK population have some sort of respiratory disease.

The lungs accomplish so much more than just the exchange of oxygen and carbon-dioxide, they also:

- Stabilise the acid and alkali balance in the body
- Defend against bacterial and other pathogenic infections
- Regulate temperature
- Eliminate toxic waste

If the lungs are not functioning properly it can have a serious effect on the whole body.

The two main underlying causes for respiratory disease are inhalation of toxic substances, in particular smoking, and infections.

The lungs accommodate a huge surface area, which is directly in contact with the outside world, in that we are directly inhaling air and other gases from our environment into the body. If any of this air contains noxious substances, they dissolve in the mucus lining of our lungs and get absorbed into the system. These toxic substances can then damage the lung surface and reduce the capacity for gas exchange. Studies show that living in cities increases considerably the risk for respiratory disease, be it asthma, lung cancer, COPD (Chronic Obstructive Pulmonary Disorder – a chronic inflammatory lung disease) or acute lower respiratory tract infections.[15]

Any infectious agents that are inhaled have direct access to the internals of the body and have to be fought off by our immune system.

CANCER

It is interesting to note that the most prevalent cancers (lung, colon, breast and prostate) arise in those areas of the body that are in contact with toxins from the environment. The colon is exposed to foods that we ingest and the breast and prostate glands are being affected by the hormone-disrupting chemicals in our environment.

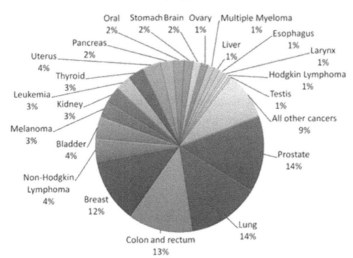

Incidence by type of cancer

What are the causes of cancer?
Many of us have been led to believe that cancer is a genetic problem – we have this potential sword of Damocles

hanging over our heads which might fall if we are unlucky. However, cancer does not work like this. The rates at which cancers are being diagnosed are such that now 1 in 2 people will get cancer at some point in their life. The conventional medical approach is to either burn the cancer cells (radiotherapy), poison the cancer cells (chemotherapy) or cut them out (surgery). The main problem with the first two approaches is that the treatment cannot discriminate between the healthy cells and the cancerous cells. For a body that is already under strain, trying to get the cancer under control, to have to cope with healthy cells being damaged cannot be a sound approach. The other method of surgery is also not ideal as you end up cutting out important areas of the body that perform a function – remember the body works as a whole and if you remove organs or tissue, there is not only the detrimental effect of having lost some or all of that organ, but also the body's stress response to this loss, which can impact the entire system.[16]

When you look at the fundamental workings of a cancer cell, the conventional approaches are missing the point. A healthy cell develops into a cancer cell due to the environment that it is exposed to; you can burn it, poison it or cut it out, but none of this changes the environment, so there is a risk that it may return, particularly when you add in the carcinogenic effects of the chemotherapy and the radiotherapy.[17]

Factors in the environment that promote cancer
- Excess insulin – from excess sugar / refined carbohydrate consumption
- Free radical damage – caused by stress, sunburn, eating excess sugar, burnt food, pollution, excessive levels of exercise, bacterial or viral infection – see Antioxidants in FOOD Chapter
- Excess oestrogen or testosterone – hormone-

disrupting chemicals in the environment, including the contraceptive pill and HRT; these excess hormones particularly drive breast, uterine and prostate cancer – see SLUDGE Chapter

- Acid / Alkali imbalance – cancer cells love an acidic environment
- Diet – consuming excessive amounts of sugar and carbohydrates and eating nutrient-deficient foods
- Psychological stress
- Environmental toxins including radiation
- Genetics – 'genes load the gun but the environment pulls the trigger'
- Virus / Bacterial Infection – preoccupies the immune system when it should be scanning for cancer cells.

A POORLY FUNCTIONING IMMUNE SYSTEM is key to the development of cancer – most of the immune system is based in the gut, so our gut health is imperative for cancer prevention. See GUT Chapter.

If we change these factors, we are removing the driving forces that can damage the DNA of a cell so that it mutates and becomes cancerous. This would have a profound effect upon cancer statistics. If you do have cancer it is really important that you don't start playing the blame game, the situation is what it is, what I wish is for you to feel empowered and know that there is something that you can do about it.

Taking your treatment and healing programme into your own hands is a courageous move. I would not presume to imagine what a diagnosis of cancer feels like; however, I have seen it many times and the fear it induces makes it very tempting to hand over control to the 'experts'. It is so much easier and more comfortable to have somebody else make all the decisions. I am also not suggesting that no one should have conventional treatment, a dual approach can work well, but I feel that it is imperative to change the environment that the cells are being exposed to, in order to ensure that you are not making it easy for the cancer to return. Most oncologists have a narrow training when it comes to cancer (much of their training is paid for by Big Pharma) and simply don't know / believe that there is any other way than chemotherapy, radiotherapy and surgery. There are multiple scientifically-based alternative approaches, and doctors need to be given the freedom to do what is best for their patients. One of my jobs when I see someone with cancer is to give them the confidence to be in charge, to do their own research, ask questions, query treatments etc. There is a whole raft of information out there that is invaluable; however, it can be confusing to sift through it all. There will always be the claims – *I healed my cancer with bicarbonate of soda / wheatgrass / juicing etc.* I am not saying that any of these do not work, they were the right thing for that individual person, everyone is different and the underlying causes of their cancer will differ. It is important that you find the right treatment for you. I suggest that you sign up with a functional medicine practitioner to help guide you through the maze. Another extremely useful resource is 'The Truth about Cancer' website set up by Ty Bollinger.

I think it would be helpful at this point to look at a few of the characteristics of a cancer cell and how it differs from a normal healthy cell.

Cancer cells love sugar
In relation to cancer, sugar consumption is key because cancer cells can only run on glucose as a fuel. A normal healthy cell can use sugar or fat. All cancer patients should be made aware of this fact – if you eat sugar or any carbohydrate-dense foods, you are providing a source of fuel for those cancer cells – sadly this information is not being passed on to

cancer patients, rarely do oncologists know about or educate their patients about diet.

Two years ago, I went to hear Sophie Sabbage talk at a local cancer centre. If you have cancer and you have not come across Sophie, I urge you to look at her work; she has written *The Cancer Whisperer*, which is hugely inspiring and empowering. I walked into this cancer centre to see a table laden with cakes and biscuits etc; one of the carers there was extolling the generosity of the families of cancer patients who had provided all of these goodies for everyone. I asked as diplomatically as possible if the cancer patients were given any kind of education about diet. The essence of the reply was that as cancer was such a tough road it was nice for the patients to have these treats. Now, I am not disputing that cancer must be a very tough road, but these patients were not even being given the information to make an informed choice. Most people who come to see me with cancer don't know any of this dietary information. Some of them are often quite frustrated, having asked their oncologist what they should be eating and having been told: 'Eat what you like, it doesn't make any difference.' Nutrition education should be an absolute priority for cancer patients in order to give them a sense of empowerment.

However, we do need to make sure that it is the right advice, I had one client being told to eat lots of sugar by a dietician because he had become cachexic (uncontrollable weight-loss due to the high metabolic rate of the cancer cells). If you are underweight eat more fat: this will fuel your body but not the cancer cells. Fat consumption also means that there is no insulin production; insulin encourages the growth of cancer cells.

Cancer cells tend to grow at a much faster rate than a healthy cell, so they have quite a voracious appetite for glucose. Let me explain how a PET scan works. These scans are done if there is suspected cancer in the body, this is where a radioactive tracer, which is bound to glucose, is injected into the body. Because the cancer cells are more greedy for the glucose, when the body is scanned the increased concentration of the radioactive material will show up. On this premise, if we were wanting to starve the cancer cells, surely we should try to remove as much glucose from the diet as possible.

If you look at the typical Western diet, that doesn't leave much – but don't panic, I can assure you that nature has provided us with plenty of vibrant health-supporting foods that won't feed cancer. Your major source of fuel will be fat.

Fat – coconut oil, olive oil, flax oil, sesame oil, pumpkin-seed oil (not sunflower oil as it is high in omega 6, which can cause inflammation), all nut oils, avocado oil and ghee. See FOOD Chapter for information on cooking with oils.

Ghee is the oil from butter with the milk solids removed; if you have cancer I would remove all sources of dairy – milk, cheese, yoghurt, butter. Dairy products have growth hormones in them which could encourage the growth of cancer.

Foods to support liver function – this is especially important if you are having chemotherapy as you need to support the detox process as much as possible.

Dark green leafy vegetables – broccoli, kale, cabbage, Brussels sprouts, watercress, rocket, spinach

Sulphurous foods – eggs, onions, garlic, leeks, parsley.

Foods to provide lots of antioxidants e.g. bright-coloured vegetables – peppers, beetroot, tomatoes, cucumber, green beans, purple cabbage. Lemons are the only fruit allowed.

Avocado

Herbs and spices, there are multiple health benefits to herbs and spices, in particular turmeric, cinnamon, rosemary, thyme, basil, sage, ginger. They will also make your food more delicious.

Protein – a small amount is helpful but keep levels low, ideally 1gm per kilo of your lean body mass. I would stick to fish, eggs, some nuts and seeds – excess protein can stimulate the mTOR pathway, which in turn encourages growth.

I know this looks like a very restricted diet but when your body goes so off-piste as to produce cancer, it requires a bit of hard graft to bring it back into balance. It is helpful to look at food in a different way – everything you ingest needs to be medicinal, until you can obtain that balance back and then you can relax the regime a bit. This way of eating should get your body burning fat as fuel rather than glucose, slightly depending on your body and how many vegetables you are eating. For information on a full ketogenic diet I recommend that you look at the work of Dr Reinwald.

Cancer cells hate oxygen, which creates an alkali environment
This is a characteristic of cancer cells discovered back in the 1930s by Otto Warburg (why is it taking so long for this to become mainstream?). Cancer cells cannot survive in the presence of high levels of oxygen. This is because high levels of oxygen create a more alkali environment and cancer cells thrive in acidic conditions. To explain this further we have to delve into a bit of chemistry again.

Water: H_2O, which makes up 50–65% of the body, can split into an H ion and an OH ion, and if there is an excess of H ions then the environment will be acidic, a surplus of OH ions then the environment will be alkali. If you create a surplus of oxygen in the body then many of the H ions will be joined by an oxygen atom, thus creating a more alkali environment.

On this premise it might be sound practice to increase oxygen levels in the body; this can be done with exercise, but many who are suffering with cancer do not have the energy or inclination to be doing lots of exercise, so I suggest that you find a local hyperbaric oxygen chamber and sit in this or sign up for some ozone therapy. Additionally ensuring that you are breathing correctly can also help – see STRESS Chapter.

There are other ways of increasing the alkalinity of the body, which ideally wants to be pH 7.2 or just above. Lots of green will help – wheatgrass, chlorella, spirulina etc; also, you can take baking soda (use the Arm & Hammer brand which does not contain aluminium) in water to increase alkalinity, 1 teaspoon in a glass of water per day. It is advisable to monitor your pH levels using pH urine sticks, which you can purchase very easily.

Above I have given you some very basic ideas of how to help balance your body and make it an inhospitable place for cancer cells; if you have cancer there is a whole lot more you can do. 'The Truth about Cancer' website is an ideal place to start and I would really recommend working alongside a functional medicine practitioner. For those who do not have cancer or who may have a history of cancer in the family, introducing the above dietary recommendations can go a long way to prevent it, alongside addressing your toxic exposure, emotional baggage and stress levels.

A word on emotions – in my experience the emotion most associated with cancer is very often anger. When I suggest this to clients they often say, 'No I don't think I am angry' but on further reflection, when the onion layers start peeling back it can often be found. Anger is just fear with attitude, and when we look more deeply there is often deep-seated fear (usually from childhood) that is being carried in the body. Depression is also viewed as a person's anger that is turned inwards against the self. I read somewhere that cancer is the body's metaphor for the extreme need to grow, which I thought was an interesting idea to be considered. It is important that the emotional element is not ignored, often one of the most challenging elements to deal with.

TYPE 2 DIABETES

To explain this issue simply, when we are consuming too much sugar and carbohydrate, the body has to produce lots of insulin, which travels around in the bloodstream getting the cells to take up the excess sugar. If insulin is constantly asking the cells to take up sugar the cells become resistant and stop taking any notice of the message. The excess sugar then gets sent to the liver where it is converted into fat and put around the middle. There are many people walking around today with skinny arms and legs and large middles, this is a sure sign that they have become insulin resistant. (I will mention here that you don't have to be overweight to have Type 2 diabetes, some bodies manage to avoid the weight gain but the cells are still insulin resistant.)

Excess fat cells around the middle, as well as being bad for you posturally, are also very harmful because they produce extra oestrogen (drives cancer, endometriosis, fibroids etc) and inflammatory cytokines which are messengers that promote inflammation. Inflammation, as discussed above, is the fire that keeps chronic disease running, so these inflammatory cytokines will exacerbate any type of disease in the body.

This is a quote from the 'Diabetes UK' website:

'More people than ever have diabetes. More people than ever are at risk of Type 2 diabetes. If nothing changes, more than five million people will have diabetes in the UK by 2025.'

Scary statistics yes, but the bit that concerns me is the 'at risk of Type 2 diabetes', as if there is *nothing* we can do about it. As with so many other chronic diseases, the medical profession are hunting for a cure, that magic pill to solve things, but we already have a cure for Type 2 diabetes. Change the diet so that you are not eating foods that require such a high level of insulin, e.g. less sugar and carbohydrate.

NEURODEGENERATIVE DISEASE – ALZHEIMER'S,
PARKINSON'S AND DEMENTIA

This is the type of disease that terrifies people the most – so many say: 'I can cope with whatever is thrown at me physically … but please don't let me lose my mind.' There is a huge fear of the indignity and humiliation of a situation where your body is still there, but you are no longer you. Relatives have to mourn the loss of their loved ones twice: firstly when cognition is so damaged that they cease to be that person, and then secondly when, god willing, the body ceases functioning. The diagnosis of dementia or Alzheimer's is also so frightening because we have all been given the message that there is nothing that can be done to stop this process of degeneration. All the billions of pounds that have been spent on trying to find a drug to fix the problem have failed. The problem is that drugs can only target one or two issues at a time and, according to Dr Dale Bredesen in his book *The End of Alzheimer's*, there are approximately 36 different factors that can be involved in the progression of these diseases. Not all of these factors will be involved in every individual, but the skill is finding out which ones are causing an imbalance and then fixing them.

Dr Bredesen states 'Alzheimer's disease can be prevented, and in many cases its associated cognitive decline can be reversed.' This is phenomenally exciting news: I was hopping up and down when I read Dr Bredesen's book.

If you are at all concerned about your memory, I urge you to read his work. Brain degeneration is a complex topic and one that is beyond the scope of this book, however, there are some important basic factors that drive brain inflammation and damage.

They are:

STRESS – stress hormones in excess can cause all sorts of damage and an excess of cortisol has been shown to harm the hippocampal cells. The hippocampus in the brain plays an important role in short-term, long-term and spatial memory – vital for navigation. The hippocampus is one of the main areas to be damaged in Alzheimer's.

LACK OF SLEEP – reduces the amount of time for cleaning out the brain.

EXPOSURE TO TOXINS – a dirty brain cannot function properly.

INFLAMMATION – this can be driven by leaky gut, chronic infection, excess sugar in the diet, toxicity, stress, postural abnormalities which cause joint damage and muscle tension etc. A useful blood test to check your levels of inflammation is to look at the C-Reactive Protein levels, this is a straightforward blood test that most GPs should be happy to do.

DIET – excess sugar and refined carbohydrates – the most inflammatory food you can eat.[18] Within the category of carbohydrate we have gluten – if you read the work of David Perlmutter, a neurologist who wrote *Grain Brain*, he shows evidence that gluten has a very large part to play in neurological disease and you don't have to be a coeliac for this to be the case. Time and time again he observes an improvement in his patients when they come off gluten.

DIGESTIVE ISSUES – firstly, if your digestion is not working properly you will not be absorbing the necessary nutrients for optimal brain health. Secondly, if you have digestive issues it usually means that your levels of gut bacteria are out of balance; there is much evidence to show that a healthy gut microbiome can reduce the risk of neurodegenerative disease.[19] See GUT Chapter.

VITAMIN D DEFICIENCY – vitamin D deficiency is correlated with cognitive decline.[20]

ESSENTIAL FAT DEFICIENCY – studies show that

not eating enough foods that contain essential fats – e.g. oily fish, nuts and seeds – increases the risk for Alzheimer's and dementia.[21]

LACK OF CHOLESTEROL – if your levels of cholesterol are too low you are more at risk of Parkinson's disease and dementia.[22]

THYROID HORMONE IMBALANCE – the thyroid controls your metabolic rate; if this is turned down too low or turned up too high both can have a profound effect upon the workings of the brain. See THYROID Chapter. Sex hormone imbalance can also affect brain function.

RAISED HOMOCYSTEINE – homocysteine is a substance that can accumulate in the body if you are not methylating properly. Methylation is a process of adding a methyl group (CH3) to DNA, and this process turns genes on and off. It happens in every single cell of our body, thousands of times a day. 'An increased plasma homocysteine level is a strong, independent risk factor for the development of dementia and Alzheimer's disease'.[23] Not only is it a risk factor for Alzheimer's, it can also indicate your risk of cardiovascular disease, cancer, hormone imbalance, mental health issues, autoimmune disease and allergies. This is something that everyone should have tested as a matter of course. If you have higher homocysteine levels, it is important to be taking increased amounts of vitamins B6, B12 and in particular folate, but they must be in the methylated form. There are specific supplements for reducing homocysteine that contain these and other nutrients.

LACK OF EXERCISE – exercise increases muscle contraction, muscle contraction increases the flow of lymph, which helps with detoxing and also boosts blood flow to bring extra nutrients and oxygen to the brain. If you don't have high blood pressure, doing inverted postures e.g. shoulder, head or handstands (or just getting your head below your heart) daily can improve your brain function as you get a good blood rush to the head.

SEDENTARY BRAIN – use it or lose it – keeping your brain active promotes a denser network of neurons and also preserves a healthy blood supply.[24] Try sudoku, crosswords, learning a new language or partaking in some of the online brain-training websites.

Many of the factors in the above list can be involved in all chronic diseases, it just depends on which is the weakest part of your body – this will be the part that starts to show symptoms first.

AUTOIMMUNE DISEASES

Autoimmunity is one category of disease that has increased considerably since I started practising ten years ago. This is where the immune system loses the ability to differentiate between self and non-self, so it starts to attack certain tissues of the body. With autoimmunity, the antibodies have been attacking tissue for years before we start to experience symptoms.

They are diseases such as:

Coeliac – where the immune system attacks the gut wall every time we eat gluten, in fact many other tissues in the body can be at risk every time a person eats gluten. Coeliac disease is a very complex condition; if you have this issue, I urge you to look at the work of Dr Tom O'Bryan.

Rheumatoid Arthritis – the immune system attacks the joints.

Hashimoto's / Graves – the immune system attacks the thyroid gland, making it underactive or overactive.

Ulcerative Colitis – the immune system attacks the wall of the colon and rectum to the point where it produces ulcers.

MS – the immune system starts to attack the myelin sheath – this is the protective cover of nerve cells in the brain and spinal cord.

In fact, there are approximately 80 different types of auto-immune disease. As our immune systems become more and more overwhelmed by our environment, they can start to attack any tissue in the body, so I don't think that the number will be stopping at 80.

Conventional medicine in its wisdom has decided that the best way to deal with these diseases is to give drugs to suppress the immune system. This may relieve symptoms; however, if you have a suppressed immune system it can't help you fight off bacterial / viral infections. I am not just talking about the proper full-blown infections that we are aware of; many of us carry low grade infections, there is no fanfare of illness but these disorders have a slow insidious effect that runs us down and makes us feel 'just not right'. A fully functioning immune system is vital to help our bodies deal with all infections that we come into contact with, in addition to eradicating cancer cells.

Again, we have to ask the question – what has upset the immune system so much that it has lost the ability to differentiate between self and non-self? As 80% of our immune system is based in the gut, this would be my first port of enquiry: is there damage to the gut wall? It is after all very delicate. Are food proteins or any substances that we are ingesting (not always technically food when you start reading the labels on food packets) leaking through the damaged gut wall and setting the immune system on red alert – if this happens on a chronic basis the immune system can become a bit trigger-happy and start attacking things that it shouldn't. See GUT Chapter for other factors that can damage the gut wall.

*

How autoimmunity works

The immune system operates by analysing the shapes of proteins to decide whether to attack or not. Proteins are made of different sequences of amino acids; there are only 22 amino acids but there are countless combinations and thus types of proteins. Many of these proteins will have similar sequences of amino acids in their make-up. This is where it can get confusing for the immune system, for example gluten and the proteins in a thyroid cell have a similar sequence of amino acids, this is why there is a much greater likelihood of people who are reacting to gluten developing autoimmune thyroid problems. Gluten is one of the main foods that can trigger autoimmunity and if you are reacting to it there is also a possibility that you are cross-reacting to other grains as well because they have similar amino acid sequences. There is a blood test (Cyrex Laboratories US) that you can get done to see if you have developed auto-antibodies to parts of your body.

One of the reasons why women are more susceptible to autoimmune diseases is that they have more oestrogen in their system than men. Oestrogen reduces the amount of T-suppressor cells. T-suppressor cells are responsible for closing the immune system down after it has responded to a foreign assault. Without these cells the immune system can go on a trigger-happy rampage around the body. Our environment is exposing us to increased levels of oestrogen, this factor is one of the reasons why autoimmunity is increasing. If you want to delve further into this topic, I recommend that you read *The Autoimmune Solution* by Amy Myers.

Whilst we are on the subject of the immune system and Covid-19 is rampaging across the world, I feel that it would be remiss of me not to share with you my advice to clients regarding this immune challenge. Firstly I would point you to the advice starting on page 33, all of these factors will affect the potency of our immune system. In addition I recommend supplementing with vitamin D3 – in a perfect world we would all have our levels tested but at this time I don't want to put the NHS under any more pressure – I advise you have 2000iu of vitamin D3 a day, especially if you are living in the northern hemisphere where we haven't seen the sun for a while. I also recommend taking 3000mg of vitamin C on a daily basis (this is not long term; once we are through the risk of infection I would drop to 1000mg a day), ideally not the fizzy sugary ones; take it in a capsule form. Additionally, zinc has been shown to inhibit the replication of Covid-19[25] so taking 30mg of zinc citrate a day will help. Make sure that you are drinking enough water and most importantly of all I recommend that people keep their spirits up; if you are having to self-isolate be in touch on the phone/computer etc. As you will read later our mental wellbeing has a very profound effect upon our immune system. If you are feeling ill then take a duvet day or even a duvet week, allow the body to do what it does best and that is to heal us.

I have covered some of the major diseases that afflict our population today and hope that you now understand that many of them have similar underlying mechanisms driving them. I want to look in more detail at some of these factors and how we can change them, but before we do that I want to explain about a vital gland and the devastating effect it can have if it is not working properly.

3

THYROID – THE ENERGY
GLAND

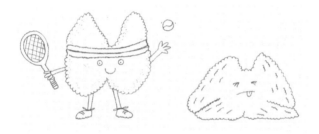

Although the pituitary gland is described as the master gland of the body, in my experience the thyroid is the one that goes wrong the most often with very far-reaching effects. Research shows that approximately 80% of the population are walking around with undiagnosed thyroid problems, particularly women, and I was one of them so the thyroid is very close to my heart – literally!

In the days before I started upon my wonderful nutrition journey, I was flying around with three small children, eating the wrong things – don't get me wrong, my diet was not particularly bad but it was not helping me in my quest to cope with a hectic life. I kept going to the doctor saying 'I know that there is something wrong, I feel as if I am walking through treacle all the time.' The doctor obligingly did blood tests, including looking at my thyroid, but always the tests kept coming back 'normal' and I went away with my heart sinking, knowing that there was something wrong but having no idea how to fix it. It just couldn't be normal to feel so exhausted, but my blood test results were saying that there was nothing the matter and I didn't want to make a fuss! It wasn't until a year later when I started to study the thyroid on my nutrition course that everything fell into place. Let me explain more.

One of the big problems with testing for thyroid issues is that the NHS, unless specifically asked for other readings (and even then they are usually reluctant as it all costs money) will only test your TSH (thyroid stimulating hormone) levels.

I think a diagram may help here:

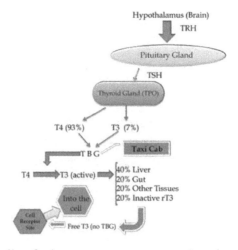

It takes all of these processes to make the thyroid hormones so they become active in the body.

As you can see TSH is not the whole thyroid story, this is what the pituitary gland produces and sends to the thyroid to tell it to work harder when general feedback reaches the brain's hypothalamus saying that thyroid hormone levels are a bit low. When thyroid hormones are low everything is on go-slow mode. As you will see from the diagram, there are many other cogs in this system that can go awry and produce symptoms of an imbalanced thyroid. Starting at the top.

There can be an imbalance in the hypothalamus – often due to chronic stress, this is one of the major factors that is pushing so many people's thyroids out of balance. Chronic stress takes the hypothalamus's eye off the ball, there is a sabre-toothed tiger to fight so TRH production goes on the back burner which means the pituitary gland does not get the TRH (thyroid releasing hormone) message.

There can be an imbalance in the pituitary so that not enough TSH (thyroid stimulating hormone) is produced – most often due to chronic stress.

The conversion of T4 (the inactive thyroid hormone) to T3 (the active form) which dictates how fast your metabolic rate goes, is not working properly. If there are high levels of cortisol (stress hormone) circulating in the body, it supresses the conversion of T4 to T3 in order to try and stop the body from burning out. This was my problem, my TSH levels were normal and so were my T4 levels; it was the conversion that was not happening.

There are raised levels of rT3 (reverse T3) – rT3 is produced when there is extreme or chronic stress occurring. This happens to try and slow the body down as it is living in high velocity fight / flight mode too much of the time, which can again lead to burn-out – basically this makes you feel exhausted so you have to slow down.

Another problem is autoimmunity, discussed in the previous chapter. In this case it is the thyroid gland that is the target and the result is an imbalance of thyroid function, be it a ramping up of the metabolic rate because too much thyroid hormone is produced, as in Graves disease, or a slowing down of function, as in Hashimoto's.

If you are getting your thyroid tested these are ideally the readings that you need to ask for:

- TSH
- Total T4
- Free T4
- Free T3
- Reverse T3
- Anti Thyroglobulin – auto-antibody
- Anti Thyroid peroxidase – auto-antibody

If your GP won't do it, it is possible to get it done privately, but I suggest that you find a good functional medicine practitioner to guide you through the process of helping to interpret results and working out the best way forward to balance the thyroid.

WHY IS THE THYROID SO IMPORTANT AND WHAT DOES IT DO?

The thyroid dictates how fast your body runs, i.e. your metabolic rate. It responds to every little nuance of your day, producing tiny amounts of thyroid hormones in order to keep everything balanced.

It profoundly impacts energy levels by increasing the rate of mitochondria – these are the little energy-generating organelles found in every cell of the body. If cellular energy is in decline that affects every tissue / organ.

If you are feeling cold, it will increase heat production.

If there is an infection to fight, it will ramp up the immune system.

It will dictate how fast food moves through your gut and how efficiently you absorb nutrients.

It is involved in providing fuel for the muscles.

It helps to control the rate and strength of the heartbeat.

It will increase the rate of breathing if there is a lack of oxygen in the tissues.

It is involved in maintaining a normal menstrual cycle and impacts libido.

It helps with quality of sleep.

If your thyroid is imbalanced it can impact every area of your body and completely kybosh your life.

One of the reasons that some people do not always improve on thyroid medication is that you take your thyroid hormone (usually in the form of T4 – thyroxine) in one dose first thing in the morning, which gives you an initial boost, but then levels of T4 can run a bit low towards the end of the day so there is not so much ability to respond to events later. Another problem with taking thyroxine, the usual thyroid medication, is that it is T4, which is the inactive hormone; it needs to be converted to T3 to have an effect on the metabolic rate but if, as I did, you have high cortisol levels, this conversion does not happen as it should.

Other factors that can affect this conversion are imbalanced gut bacteria – the beneficial bacteria produce intestinal sulfatase, which helps to convert about 20% of T4 to T3. We also need to make sure that we have good stocks of selenium, zinc, vitamin D and vitamin A, all of these nutrients vital for this conversion to occur. It is possible to get thyroid medication in the form of T3 but it is more expensive and many doctors are reluctant to prescribe it. With my thyroid issue I started taking some bio-identical (not synthetic) T4 and T3 but it still didn't have the effect of improving my energy levels. After a little while I had to admit that my thyroid issue was purely down to stress and I could try and fix it with T4 and T3 till the cows came home but my body in a bid to prevent burn-out was not going to play ball. Since then, I have been working on my adrenals and supporting thyroid function with nutrients and things are now more balanced, but it is something that I need to keep under surveillance.

If your thyroid is under-functioning – this is hyp<u>O</u>thyroid – these are the typical symptoms that you might experience:

- Lack of energy, generally feeling sluggish physically and mentally
- Hypersensitive to cold, in particular cold hands and feet
- Increased susceptibility to infections – colds and viruses etc.
- Constipation
- Digestive issues
- Muscle cramps
- Hypoglycemia – signs of low blood sugar levels: dizzy, shaky, irritable, fatigue, loss of concentration if you don't eat regularly
- Dry skin and hair
- Inability to lose weight and gaining weight easily
- Hair loss – in particular the outer third of the eyebrow
- Puffy face
- Needing more sleep than usual
- Depression
- Slow wound healing
- Hoarse voice
- Often feeling like you have a frog in your throat
- Raised cholesterol levels
- Goitre – visible swelling of the neck where the thyroid gland has started to enlarge.
- Gallstones
- Heart palpitations

- Night sweats
- Insomnia

This is not an exhaustive list and you may not experience all of these symptoms but even a few may indicate that it would be worth investigating your thyroid function.

If your thyroid is over-functioning – HypERthyroid – these are the type of symptoms that you might experience:

- Heart palpitations
- Increased pulse rate, even when resting
- Inability to gain weight, often with an increased appetite
- Difficulty concentrating
- Inward trembling
- Hand tremor
- Night sweats
- Intolerance to heat
- Insomnia
- Feeling wired
- Feeling over-emotional
- Feeling anxious
- Fatigue
- Hoarse voice
- Often feeling like you have a frog on your throat
- Goitre – visible swelling of the neck where the thyroid gland has started to enlarge

The confusing thing is, when your thyroid is out of balance it can swing from hypERthyroid to hypOthyroid and back again so you may be experiencing symptoms from both of these lists. This swinging about can also make it confusing with regard to blood tests because you may get the blood tested when you are in hypO or hypER state or somewhere in the middle.

Other things that can affect thyroid function

Contraceptive pill or HRT – excess oestrogen increases thyroid binding globulin (TBG) – see diagram, this is a protein that transports the thyroid hormones around the body. Whilst the thyroid hormones are bound by TBG, they are inactive, if there is too much TBG then the thyroid hormone will be trapped and it can't enter the cell and take effect.

Close together pregnancies – this I think was a trigger for me: I had three children in just over three years. Pregnancy is hard work for the mother's body and it requires the metabolic rate to increase slightly. Scans show that the thyroid actually increases in size by up to 15% during pregnancy. I am not saying don't have your babies close together, I highly recommend it from a family dynamics point of view, but be aware that your body will need some extra nurturing if you are asking it to work so hard for you.

Gut health – the correct balance of good gut bacteria for conversion of T4 to T3 is important, also the health of the gut wall, if the gut wall is a bit leaky (see GUT Chapter) it then sets the stage for autoimmune thyroid diseases like Graves (hypERthyroid) and Hashimoto's (HypOthyroid).

Liver function – as you will see from the diagram 40% of T4 is converted into T3 in the liver, and if your liver is being overworked by exposure to our toxic environment then this conversion will not happen efficiently.

Iodine levels – many people are deficient in iodine; however, a word of caution – if you have autoimmune thyroid disease, taking iodine can make things worse. I recommend that you ask your GP to check your iodine levels. Other elements that have a similar molecular structure to iodine and so can plug into the iodine receptors on the thyroid and affect function are flouride and chlorine. I would always recommend using fluoride-free toothpaste and finding a pool that uses alternatives to chlorine, or even better swimming in the sea / lakes / rivers.

Nutrient deficiencies – lack of of selenium, zinc, vitamin D and vitamin A and iodine as well as…

Essential fatty acids – oily fish and nuts and seeds.

Iron – one of the most difficult nutrients for our body to break down and absorb. It is important that iron levels are tested before supplementation because having excess iron in the system can increase inflammation and cause damage. It is also important to ensure that the form of iron that is being supplemented is correct; many doctors give out iron sulphate which has a very strong chemical bond between the iron and sulphate so that the digestive system struggles to break this bond in order to absorb the iron. It is also more likely to upset the gut in this form; easier forms of iron to absorb are iron citrate or fumerate and it is helpful to always take vitamin C with the iron, at least 1000mg to help with absorption. Doctors often recommend having orange juice with an iron supplement to provide vitamin C but as you will read later I am not a fan of fruit juice.

In my experience testing for thyroid issues is problematic because with a blood test you are getting a snapshot of what is going on in the body, not an idea over time. For me I rely more and more upon the list of symptoms of imbalanced thyroid function and then look at all the factors that can affect the thyroid in order to try and balance things up. The one test that is accurate is testing for antibodies to the thyroid; if you have antibodies there is an autoimmune situation that needs to be dealt with. This means that gut health becomes a priority.

To finish I would like to touch on the emotional element of the thyroid. The thyroid is in the throat area and many people with thyroid problems have throat issues, hoarse voice or feeling like you often have a frog in your throat. It can be useful to look at whether you are expressing yourself and your needs honestly, I asked one client with serious thyroid issues this question, and she paused and then said 'How long have you got?' She was involved in a marriage where for decades she had constantly had to suppress her emotions, keep the peace and not express her needs fully. Again, I come back to the idea that our body speaks a language, the symptoms that it expresses are reminding us that our environment needs to change, be it emotionally or physically. Interestingly it is more women than men who experience thyroid issues.

4

CONVENTIONAL MEDICINE VERSUS FUNCTIONAL MEDICINE

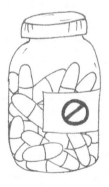 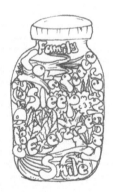

'The doctor of the future will give no medicine, but will instruct his patient in the care of the human frame, in diet, and in the cause and prevention of disease.'
— Thomas Edison

This is a really hard chapter to write because I don't want to annoy / upset all of the great doctors and other medical staff who are practising conventional medicine and are doing their very best to make their patients better. However, not all medical practitioners work in the same way. On my travels as a Nutritional Therapist I have come across a whole spectrum. At one end of the scale there are the compassionate, sensitive and respectful medical staff who are prepared to think outside the box, spend extra time with their patients and are aware of the limitations of their approach. I once had a conversation with a doctor during a consultation regarding my own thyroid health about how frustrating it was for me that conventional doctors and people like myself couldn't work alongside each other. I asked him why he thought this was and he replied 'It is a mixture of fear and ignorance on our behalf.' I could have hugged him for his honesty and humility. At the other end of the scale there are those practitioners with their blinkers firmly in place who are not prepared to change the status quo. These practitioners maintain their position of power and I have clients who are scared to question any of the treatments that they are being prescribed or even be truthful about their search for another more natural approach to healing. In these cases, there is no respect for the patient as an individual, the doctor in question has attained 'god-like' status, which is often exacerbated by the staff around him / her (not so many hers but that is another story). My mission is not to beat up on those doctors who truly believe in their craft, but to empower you the reader to ask questions – will this treatment / medication really solve the underlying cause of my ailment? The evidence that I see for those with chronic disease is that pills are not the answer.

This client is an example of many I see:
David, who was in his eighties, came to see me because he had just been diagnosed as diabetic, on top of this issue he had high blood pressure, an irregular heartbeat, IBS, prostate issues, raised cholesterol and asthma. His body was really

shouting at him and for me this was a huge challenge. These medical issues do not happen overnight and had probably been brewing in his system for decades. I was going to have to persuade him to change some habits of a lifetime, quite literally. The hospital dietitian had recommended that he should eat more white bread and bananas to help stabilise his blood sugar. Now it doesn't take a Nutritional Therapist to know that this advice doesn't make sense. David was also taking 12 different medications, 2 for asthma, 4 for blood pressure, 1 for irregular heartbeat, a blood thinner, a statin to reduce cholesterol, acid reflux medication, medication for his IBS, drugs for prostate issues and just to top it off he had been advised to take regular paracetamol to reduce general pain. On researching the above cocktail of meds it was not difficult to find information stating that two of the medications that he had been given should not be taken together as it could produce a dangerously low heart rate.

The above situation is not uncommon: patients keep going back to the doctor with more and more symptoms and so are prescribed more and more medications because this is the only tool in the box that our doctors have.

Over time, the way that medicine is practised has changed beyond recognition; if we look back, initially much of it involved appeasing angry spirits who were thought to have vented their spleen on a particular individual who had 'strayed' from the path. Herbs and energy medicine were the order of the day for those brave souls who were prepared to reveal their healing gifts at the risk of being burned at the stake. Then Hippocrates (460–370 BC) came along and began the process of freeing medicine from superstition. He looked at the body as a whole being rather than dividing it up into different parts and believed that the symptoms of disease were caused by the body's reaction to imbalance and that the physician's role was to try and restore that balance. The adage attributed to Hippocrates of 'First do no harm' is something that all modern physicians should bear in mind before getting out their prescription pads.

The Hippocratic Oath, which doctors officially took until 1948, talks about being aware of overtreatment, that 'warmth, sympathy and understanding might outweigh the surgeon's knife or the chemist's drug', that a physician does 'not treat a fever chart, a cancerous growth, but a sick human being, whose illness may affect the person's family and economic stability'. It is important to be able to say 'I know not' and pass a patient on to the skills of another and most importantly to prevent disease wherever they can, as prevention is surely preferable to cure.

Sadly, in my experience, and in that of so many clients that I see, conventional medicine is failing us. Much of the problem boils down to lack of funds and a powerful pharmaceutical industry. A GP has a ten-minute appointment with a sick patient, not much time to get to the underlying cause of a symptom or take the time to really listen to what is going on in a patient's life. GPs have to forgo working with the body and learning to understand what the symptoms mean and instead give something to suppress those symptoms. In the short term it is quick and cheap but in the long term far more expensive and detrimental to our body and the health system.

Another problematic element is that conventional medicine is based upon Newtonian physics, the realm of the physical, you need to be able to view it under a microscope for it to be real, but this paradigm leaves out the enormous field of quantum physics and how energy affects the body. This is what so many complementary therapies are based upon and for some it can all be a bit woo-woo. Take an MEG; as opposed to an EEG, an MEG measures the electrical activity in the brain. It measures the energy field of the brain, the electrodes are not attached to the head, they are measuring the energy that extends beyond the realm of the physical body. If you are standing within this field it can affect you. I will look more into this concept in later chapters.

This physical-only sticking-plaster approach, giving the patient a pill that will suppress the symptoms often means that other symptoms are created elsewhere. Our body is communicating with us all of the time, and if we put our fingers in our ears and take medication our body cannot heal itself. Surely there must be a way for us to treat chronic disease that makes the body stronger and more vibrant, rather than introducing drugs that cover up the symptoms and inflict increasing amounts of side effects.

Conventional medicine is not all bad news, there are outstanding doctors out there who are truly doing a phenomenal job in acute situations. There are times when conventional medicine is the only and the very best option. If you have an acute problem, an accident, heart attack, stroke or organ failure – get yourself to A&E, the best place to stabilise the body. However, going forward the drugs are unlikely to heal, that is what the body does best but it will need good nutrition and a nurturing environment to do so. Most disease that we see around us today is chronic and conventional medicine is simply approaching it with the wrong tools in the box.

When you look at how conventional medicine works, it seems quite a sensible approach to divide the body up into different departments and study those areas in detail. If you have a heart problem you go and see a cardiologist, if you have hormone issues you see an endocrinologist or if you have cancer you see an oncologist. However, bodies don't work like this, everything works together and if there is a problem in one part it can impact anywhere else. The communication system in our body is phenomenal: with our cardiovascular system, substances are transported all the way around the body in approximately one minute; with our nerves, messages can be delivered at speeds ranging from a positively snail-like 20m per second to 100m per second, and then there is the information that is carried via energy in the meridian lines. There are no secrets in the body, all cells know what the other cells are up to, it is a hotbed of gossip and chatter.

In contrast to conventional medicine, functional medicine treats the body as a whole being. It treats the person and not the disease, looking at all of the systems that may be out of balance.

These systems are:
- Body Rhythm / Clock
- Oxidative Stress and Inflammation
- Hormones
- Acid and Alkali
- Neurotransmitters – Brain Chemicals
- Mitochondria – Energy Production
- Immune
- Detoxification
- Digestion
- Musculoskeletal
- Emotional

The kind of questions that I would be asking when I see a client are:

Is your body clock in balance – are you getting good-quality sleep and bouncing out of bed in the morning?

Do you have random aches and pains, this could be due to high levels of inflammation or the energy systems not producing energy in the right way so they then have to resort to anaerobic respiration (the way that we breathe when we are doing hard exercise). This type of respiration creates lactic acid, making your muscles stiff and sore. If your joints ache perhaps your liver is not detoxing properly and storing the toxins in the joints till it can deal with them at a later date.

Are your digesting your food properly? You might be eating a fantastic diet but if your body can't break it down and absorb it properly then you will be nutrient-deficient with all the problems that this entails.

Gut problems can also lead to imbalances in hormones, detoxing, mood (we make the majority of our brain chemicals in the gut) and immune issues.

What is going on for the client emotionally: is there some trauma from childhood, an unhappy marriage, a high-stress job or just life grinding them down.

Clients come through my door with a multitude of different combinations of the above, this is what makes my work so compelling and challenging. It is my job to create a safe space for them to tell their stories, which can range from simple physical symptoms to disclosing deep-seated trauma. In David's case most of his systems were out of balance, including the emotional as he had lost his wife the year before.

Keeping these systems balanced is the underlying premise of functional medicine; it talks about bio-individuality, it treats the person, not the disease, because the causes of the same disease can be very different in different people. Let me give you an example. Someone walks through my door with depression; from a functional medicine point of view that depression may be being caused by any or all of the following issues, but it is unlikely to be just one factor or an anti-depressant deficiency:

Diet lacking in nutrients for healthy brain function and production of neurotransmitters (brain chemicals which affect mood and motivation).

Digestive issues – even though the person is eating a good diet they are not breaking their food down properly and absorbing it.

Digestive tract problems – the majority of our neurotransmitters are made in the gut, if this is not functioning properly the neurotransmitters can be out of balance.

Hormone imbalance – be it sex hormones, oestrogen, progesterone, testosterone or an imbalanced thyroid function.

Excess levels of toxic chemicals in the body affecting the normal balance of brain function.

Taking medication, such as Roaccutane[26] (used to treat acne in teenagers), anti-depressants,[27] corticosteroids[28] (given to people with inflammation and autoimmune disorders), Ritalin[29] (given to thousands of children with Attention Deficit Hyperactivity Disorder), statins[30] and acid reflux[31] medication.

Any form of stress / trauma – stress involves the disruption of most physiological mechanisms in the body.

Insomnia – see SLEEP Chapter for details.

Musculoskeletal imbalance – poor posture and muscle tension can have a profound effect on the overall workings of the body. If you are not sitting, standing or generally moving correctly this leads to muscle tension and pain as the muscles try to compensate for a skeleton that is out of line. In the spine, the vertebra can become misaligned which not only causes more structural and muscular issues but also affects the nerves and blood vessels running from the spine. These nerves run to every part of the body, so for example if you have a problem with the Cervical 8 vertebra in your neck you could have problems with your hand and finger function / mobility. If you have an issue at Thoracic 6 you could have breathing and lung difficulties or with Sacral 3 there could be bladder issues. When we are busy and possibly tired, maintaining good posture is a challenge, but failure to do so can lead to so much more than just sore joints and muscles. Amy Cuddy's popular TED talk from 2012 explains how your posture can have a direct impact upon your mindset.

Imbalanced immune system – often stemming from gut problems that lead to excess inflammation in the body.

Genetic predisposition – remember our genetics are not necessarily our destiny. There is research going on currently that shows even healthy genes can act as if they are mutated, if they are exposed to an adverse environment.

Lack of physical movement – this makes it hard for the body to oxygenate and detox.

Lack of being outside in nature – see SPIRIT Chapter.

As you can see there are many reasons for a body to produce symptoms of depression, I hope throughout this book to explain to you how all of the above can lead to a sick body. To ascertain the causes of depression in a person does not just take 10 minutes and it can rarely be fixed with a pill. I have the luxury of a couple of hours with a client so we can really start digging and exploring. Sometimes it requires further testing but there are always things that we can start working on straight away.

Even as far back as the 1800s it was recognised that medication was not the solution to ill health: 'If the whole material medica, as now used, could be sunk to the bottom of the sea, it would be all the better for mankind – and all the worse for the fishes' (Oliver Wendell Holmes Senior). Unfortunately, we have a very powerful pharmaceutical industry with a huge interest in the bottom line, which drives this pill-popping mentality.

Let's take statins for example, one of the most widely prescribed drugs in the world. In 2010 a certain statin drug (Let's call it Lo-chol – I am keen to not be sued from here till kingdom come) made $13 billion for its creators. Whilst statins prevent your liver from making so much cholesterol they also prevent it from making a vital protective substance called Coenzyme Q10, which helps muscle function – your heart, being one of the most vitally important muscles in the body, needs adequate levels of this nutrient (in Canada if you are prescribed statins the label clearly states the dangers of CoQ10 depletion and advises supplementation). If your heart is low on CoQ10 you are more likely to have a heart attack.

Professor Harumi Okuyama in his study *Statins stimulate atherosclerosis and heart failure: pharmacological mechanisms*[32] stated that 'the epidemic of heart failure and atherosclerosis that plagues the modern world may paradoxically be aggravated by the pervasive use of statin drugs.'

In a meta-analysis of 11 trials from 2010,[33] the conclusion was that there was no value in statins preventing death in patients who had never had a heart attack, yet doctors are continuing to encourage vast numbers of patients to take them.

There are even moves to recommend that everyone over 50 takes statins as a precaution – think of the damage to all of those bodies, not to mention the profits for the pharmaceutical companies.

Most medications come with a large piece of paper, folded up tightly in the box, listing all the side effects of that particular drug. This is information (like lengthy terms and conditions) that people quite understandably rarely bother to read. For starters they are often written with lots of medical jargon that most of us don't understand and we have been brought up to believe that pills can make us better.

Below, as an example, is the list of side effects taken straight from the 'Lo-chol' statin drug website – I urge you to read it, it is only just over a page!

Lo-chol can cause serious side effects. These side effects have happened only to a small number of people. Your doctor can monitor you for them. These side effects usually go away if your dose is lowered or Lo-Chol is stopped. These serious side effects include:

Muscle problems. Lo-chol can cause serious muscle problems that can lead to kidney problems, including kidney failure. You have a higher chance for muscle problems if you are taking certain other medicines with Lo-chol.

Liver problems. Your doctor should run blood tests to check your liver before you start taking Lo-chol and if you have symptoms of liver problems while you take Lo-chol. Call your doctor right away if you have the following symptoms of liver problems:

feel tired or weak

loss of appetite

upper belly pain

dark amber colored urine

yellowing of your skin or the whites of your eyes

Call your doctor right away if you have:

muscle problems like weakness, tenderness, or pain that happens without a good reason, especially if you also have a fever or feel more tired than usual. This may be an early sign of a rare muscle problem.

muscle problems that do not go away even after your doctor has advised you to stop taking Lo-chol. Your doctor may do further tests to diagnose the cause of your muscle problems.

allergic reactions including swelling of the face, lips, tongue, and / or throat that may cause difficulty in breathing or swallowing which may require treatment right away.

nausea and vomiting.

passing brown or dark-colored urine.

you feel more tired than usual.

your skin and whites of your eyes get yellow.

stomach pain.

allergic skin reactions.

In clinical studies, patients reported the following common side effects while taking Lo-chol: diarrhoea, upset stomach, muscle and joint pain, and alterations in some laboratory blood tests.

The following additional side effects have been reported with Lo-chol:

tiredness, tendon problems, memory loss, and confusion.

Talk to your doctor or pharmacist if you have side effects that bother you or that will not go away.

These are not all the side effects of Lo-chol. Ask your doctor or pharmacist for a complete list.

I am now a rather nerdy reader of these documents, partly because I firstly need to know when clients are taking these medications how it is affecting their body so that I can support it with a view to damage limitation. Secondly due to a morbid fascination that the drug companies can get away with producing medication that can cause so many problems.

When patients go to see a doctor there is an expectation that they will come away with a prescription, to be sent away empty-handed with some advice on diet and lifestyle may not be what everyone is expecting or wanting. This issue was encountered by Dr Chris van Tulleken with some people in his documentary 'The Doctor Who gave up Drugs'. Let's face it, if you could take a pill to solve the underlying problem of your symptoms rather than having to do some homework on diet and lifestyle, I know which one I'd go for, but sadly mother nature doesn't work like that.

Going back to 'Lo-chol' and why statins don't help, cholesterol is absolutely vital for life; it makes up a substantial percentage of each and every cell membrane, and if your cell membranes are deficient in cholesterol they will not function properly. This means that nutrients do not enter the cell so efficiently or toxic waste is not excreted properly. A quarter of the body's cholesterol is found in the brain – one of the major side effects of taking statins is memory loss. In his book *Lipitor: Thief of Memory*, Duane Graveline a former astronaut and aerospace medical research scientist, charts his own alarming experiences of taking the drug, where within 6 weeks he failed to recognise his wife.

In the documentary *Statin Nation: The Great Cholesterol Cover-Up* the neurosurgeon Dr Natasha Campbell-McBride stated: 'The last thing you want to do is to interfere with the level of cholesterol in your body. Whatever level you have is the right level – don't mess around with it!'

Why would a doctor with years of study and training prescribe us something that has the potential to make us sick? The answer lies in the way that training is delivered: paradigms take a very long time to shift, lack of awareness is not proof of lack of evidence and in the words of Max Planck, a Nobel Prize winner in 1918, 'A new scientific truth does not triumph by convincing its opponents and making them see the light, but rather because its opponents eventually die, and a new generation grows up that is familiar with it.'

We have a pharmaceutical industry who are heavily involved in the training of medical students. It is not in their interest that new more enlightened ways of looking at the body become mainstream.

If you are on statins don't panic, start taking some Co-enzyme Q10, follow the guidelines in this book for at least 4 months before talking to your doctor about reducing / stopping your medication, but be aware many doctors do not know this information so they may be reluctant. This is when I would recommend you taking charge, do the research and make your own decision, it is after all your body.

CHOLESTEROL TESTS

Your cholesterol level is a very poor predictor of heart disease, and the majority of people who have heart attacks have 'normal' cholesterol levels.[34] I am sure you are aware of 'good' HDL and 'bad' LDL cholesterol. I have seen cholesterol results where the HDL is high which is a good thing but it raises the overall cholesterol count and patients are then being put on statins! If you want to test for your risk of heart disease you would be much better off getting readings for:

Fibrinogen – helps your blood to clot – raised levels show that you are more likely to get clots in the bloodstream, which could lead to heart attack / stroke.

C-Reactive Protein – tells us how much inflammation there is in the body.

HbA1C – how much sugar you have been consuming and whether it is sticking to your red blood cells.

Triglycerides – if we are consuming too much sugar / carbohydrate the liver will produce excess triglycerides, this is associated with the development of plaque, which blocks the blood vessels.

Homocysteine – as discussed in the second chapter there is a strong correlation between raised homocysteine levels and increased cardiovascular disease.[35]

Uric Acid – if uric acid levels are raised it indicates a chronic inflammatory state which is a major underlying cause of all cardiovascular disease.

Liver Function – the liver cleans the blood that the heart has to pump around, toxic blood creates inflammation.

If any of these are out of balance then it would be a good idea to start following the advice on page 261.

Generally, the main culprit in our diet that raises cholesterol levels is excess sugar / carbohydrate consumption.

One other 'popular' group of medications that I would like to look is are anti-anxiety / antidepressants. It is estimated that 16% of the population in the UK is taking medication for this issue, but those numbers only represent the people who are asking for help. There are three main types of medication used for this problem – anti-depressants, be-ta-blockers and benzodiazepines. I understand that in acute situations these medications can literally be a life-saver, giving a patient breathing space to try and get back on track. However, they are not a long-term solution and generally they suppress our emotion, and emotion that is unexpressed does damage in the body. Once people are put on this medication, many doctors are not keen to let patients come off them. I have clients that have been on them for years, wanting to come off, but terrified if they do that they will have rebound symptoms. There is generally no help and support being provided for them to do so. These medications often have damaging side effects.

SIDE EFFECTS OF ANTI-DEPRESSANTS – feeling agitated, shaky, anxious or depressed, feeling or being sick, indigestion and stomach aches, diarrhoea or constipation, loss of appetite, dizziness, poor sleep, headaches, low sex drive, difficulty achieving orgasm or maintaining an erection, increased risk of suicide in teenagers.

SIDE EFFECTS OF BETA-BLOCKERS – dizziness, tiredness, blurred vision, cold hands and feet, slow heartbeat, diarrhoea and nausea, poor sleep, loss of libido and difficulties maintaining an erection, depression.

SIDE EFFECTS OF BENZODIAZEPINES – drowsiness, dizziness, weakness, poor balance, depression, headache, loss of orientation, confusion, irritability, aggression and memory impairment.

Recently there have been some alarming studies done concluding that the pharmaceutical companies are being selective about the results of trials that are published. The study 'Selective publication of antidepressant trials and its influence on apparent efficacy'[36] showed that 36 out of 37 studies where the results were favourable to the drug were published, whereas only 3 out of 36 trials were published where the results were not favourable.

Conclusion – 'We cannot determine whether the bias observed resulted from a failure to submit manuscripts on the part of authors and sponsors, from decisions by journal editors and reviewers not to publish, or both. Selective reporting of clinical trial results may have adverse consequences for researchers, study participants, health care professionals, and patients.'

This situation sadly does not only apply to antidepressants – it can be seen happening across the board.

THE QUESTION OF GENETICS

If we then bring into the equation all of the different genetic mutations that each and every one of us has, our bodies will process these drugs differently, with a wide range of results. It means that when a person is given a pill for the first time it is an experiment. The doctor does not know how each individual is going to react, but it is a risk that conventional medicine is prepared to take. I am not saying that these drugs do not help some of the time but my concern is that people continue to take them long term, when providing a more nurturing environment would be far more beneficial and empowering.

One more issue with our conventional medical system that I would like to raise with you is blood tests and reference ranges. Reference ranges are sets of values that are used by doctors to see if a body is out of balance. Unfortunately, these reference ranges are calculated by taking an average of levels from people tested in the previous year. The problem with this is that, if you work on the premise that most people who visit the doctor to get their bloods taken are not on top form, it would make sense surely to rethink those levels if we want to aim for optimal health.

We are all biochemically individual, optimal levels for one person may not be optimal levels for another, and substances in the bloodstream will fluctuate from day to day, even hour to hour depending upon what your environment is throwing at you. White-coat syndrome is a perfect example – patients go to the local surgery or hospital, have their blood pressure taken, and are quite understandably a little on edge by being in that situation, then voilà, their blood pressure is up; next thing they know, they are being advised to take blood pressure medication. I would always recommend, if this happens to you, that you purchase a blood pressure monitor (approx £20) or see if the doctor's surgery will loan you one and then get an average of your blood pressure readings at home when you are more relaxed. If you have high blood pressure you can very often reduce this by taking magnesium (see FOOD Chapter), making sure that you are not dehydrated and doing breathing exercises to calm your body so that it is not scanning for the sabre-toothed tiger all of the time.

Lastly I would like to end with the most commonly prescribed medication, consumed worldwide in vast quantities on a daily basis. NSAIDS – non-steroidal anti-inflammatory drugs – basically painkillers. There is evidence to show that NSAIDS increase our risk of having a heart attack[37] but it is also general knowledge in the conventional medical world that NSAIDS lead to damage of the gut wall.[38] Very often if a patient is prescribed painkillers, they will also be prescribed something to protect the gut; these second medications are acid suppressants, which prevent your stomach from making so much acid. See GUT Chapter for the damaging effects of taking acid suppressants. I often find that in practice, a client has been put on one medication to ameliorate the effects of another. We cannot blame our doctors, they are only trying to help but they only have pills to offer and until they can offer advice on changes in lifestyle and nutrition, this situation is unlikely to change. My heart sang when I watched Dr Rangan Chatterjee's TV programme *Doctor in the House*; he is doing an outstanding job raising awareness and is now training up medical students in lifestyle medicine, but it is the tip of the iceberg and will be a long time before everyone is benefiting from GPs who are trained this way.

We are living in a pill-popping culture, our children taught that everything can be 'solved' with a pill. People pop painkillers at the slightest sign of a headache or muscle twinge and we are recommended to give our babies and young children Calpol at the slightest sign of a problem. Children today are given 3 times the amount of medication as they were 40 years ago when I was a child. Our bodies are speaking to us and they are not asking for painkillers or anti-pyretics (meds to reduce a temperature). A temperature is the body's natural way of trying to kill off an infection, and by suppressing it with medication we are very likely to prolong that infection. Re headaches, very often a headache can be solved with a glass of water and a 10-minute quiet sit-down. Muscle pain is most often due to tension in the body – where is that tension coming from? Did we overdo it in the gym, do we have a work colleague who is draining us, what is our posture like at work, are our muscles deficient in nutrients or are we setting unrealistic goals for ourselves? There could be a multitude of reasons; the skill is working out what they are.

If you are on medication, it is important that you are gentle with your body and listen to it. My suggestion is that you work with the ideas in this book for a few months before approaching your doctor to discuss reducing / stopping your medication. This way you will have got your body into a better place and more able to cope with the physiological change of less or no drugs.

I also understand that there are people with more serious health conditions for which medication is necessary; however, in these situations diet and lifestyle changes should *always* be included in the treatment protocol. The underlying principles that I will lay out in this book will be of benefit to everyone, after which it can then be decided if and what medication is really necessary. The important thing is to research your condition, get knowledgeable about these medications so that you can make an informed decision. Where there is a complex medical issue, I would always recommend to work with a functional medicine practitioner who can look at all of your body systems and see what needs supporting. However, there is nothing stopping you from adopting the basic principles in this book to see how much improvement you can achieve yourself. Go gently, a sick body that has got to the stage of showing symptoms has probably been ill for a while, possibly decades, so don't go making lots of major changes all in one go. It is also important to be aware that when a body starts healing it can give you more symptoms, e.g. when you give up coffee and you get a stonking headache. This is where it is often very helpful to have a functional medicine practitioner working alongside to guide you through this healing journey.

Forgive me if you have found this chapter rather alarming; the problem is, in order to make change we have to shout loud about things that are being swept under the carpet, otherwise the status quo will never change.

Next time your body throws a symptom at you, I respectfully suggest that for long-term benefit you would be much better off to stop and try to work out what it is trying to tell you. Yes, this approach takes a little longer and requires a bit more effort. However, in the long term your body will go on working far longer and more efficiently if you listen to it and take steps to resolve the underlying causes.

The sickness of our bodies
Shows bruising in our souls
For mind and heart and spirit
Should be treated as a whole

'In the Dreaming' by Mary Sheepshanks

5

IT'S ALL ABOUT SEX
(HORMONES)

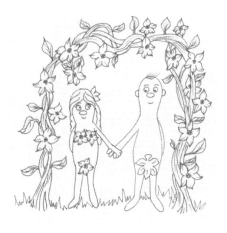

Sex hormones can have a profound effect on the wellbeing of both men and women, and when they are out of balance the symptoms produced can really make life challenging. There seems to be a growing number of people with sex hormone imbalances and the reason is mostly due to hormone-disrupting chemicals in our environment. If you also have some unhelpful genetic mutations on the liver detox pathways that process these hormones, as I do, then along with a bit of stress thrown in you have a perfect storm for hormone imbalance.

For women before menopause, I mostly see a situation where the levels of oestrogen are too high, they have become oestrogen dominant compared to the other sex hormones, progesterone and testosterone. Many chemicals in the environment that we are exposed to contain xeno-oestrogens, which are chemical forms of oestrogen, they are more potent than our own natural forms. Xeno-oestrogens plug into the hormone receptors on our cell walls and exert a powerful oestrogen-like effect. See SLUDGE Chapter.

Below are the signs that you may have too much oestrogen in your system.

- Breast tenderness
- Migraines / headaches
- Mood swings, irritability and depression
- Tiredness
- Allergies[39]
- Gallstones
- Infertility and miscarriage
- Heavy lengthy, painful periods – including clots
- Endometriosis
- Yeast overgrowth – thrush / candida
- Fibroids
- Ovarian cysts
- Polycystic ovaries
- Fibrocystic breast disease
- Brain fog and memory issues
- Low libido
- Thyroid issues
- Breast and prostate cancer

Too much oestrogen in the system, coming from the environment, is one of the main drivers of the rising rates of breast and prostate cancer. When it comes to chemical forms of oestrogen, they do not just affect women, they also affect men. Excess oestrogen in men encourages testosterone to convert to DHT (dihydrotestosterone) which is a super-charged version of testosterone and encourages the cells of the prostate gland to grow unnecessarily.

CASE STUDY – HELEN

Helen came to see me aged 36 having had heavy periods for much of her life. Her heavy periods started at 11 and she was often anaemic. Her periods had got to the stage now where they were completely debilitating, extremely heavy with large clots and severe cramping. She felt totally exhausted and 'lousy' with headaches for the day before her period and the first few days of it starting. She often had to curl up into a ball in bed with the pain and generally felt hungover (even though not drinking) had tender sore cramping muscles, stiff aching joints and her digestive symptoms were general bloating, cramping and unreliable bowel movements. Finally, as if this was not enough for one person to be dealing with, her sleep was really disrupted, she would get off OK but then wake about 2ish in the morning with her brain whirring.

Most of these symptoms pointed me towards a picture of oestrogen dominance. In order to help Helen's body process this excess oestrogen, it was important to remove as many oestrogenic items from her environment as possible. Making Helen aware of the list below meant that she could do her best to avoid any excess sources.

- Plastics – water bottles (especially those that sit in a hot car leaching even more xeno-oestrogens into the water) and packaging around food, especially if the food has a fat content – think of that cheese wrapped in clingfilm.
- Water – contains levels of oestrogen from so many women taking the contraceptive pill.

- Toiletries
- Pesticides
- Herbicides
- Fire-retardant treated fabrics
- Canned food
- Non-stick cookware
- Cleaning products
- Till receipts on thermal paper[40]
- Ink cartridges / toner

See SLUDGE Chapter for more details on environmental toxins.

Additionally, it was important to support Helen's liver function as the liver deals with excess hormones. I also recommended a supplement called DIM (Diindolylmethane) which specifically supports the detox pathway in the liver that deals with oestrogen.

Next we looked at Helen's digestive symptoms as gut flora and digestive function can have a huge impact upon the processing of hormones. A comprehensive stool analysis showed that Helen had a range of pathogenic bacteria in her gut which we needed to deal with. Pathogenic bacteria can unpackage oestrogen that has been packaged by the liver and leave it free for reabsorption. We balanced her gut bacteria by using a range of herbal anti-bacterials and also tightened up her diet so that she was not eating lots of foods that feed the pathogenic bacteria, e.g. sugar and carbs. We also introduced lots of foods to feed the good bacteria (see GUT Chapter).

It was also vital that we addressed Helen's stress levels and helped to balance her adrenal function. If your body is producing excess stress hormones this can impact the balance of your sex hormones. See below, how many of the major hormones are all connected. If the body is having to put all its effort into producing cortisol (see the second pathway), then the other hormones are going to become out of balance.

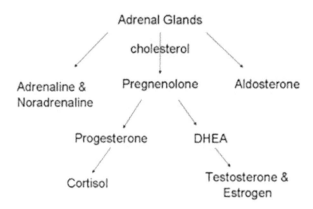

Within 2 months Helen had contacted me after having her first 'normal period' for many years – no clotting, no pain, no headaches, all her niggly muscle pains and joint aches had cleared up. She said 'It is like magic, I feel like I have been given a completely new body.' This is a great example of the body's incredible ability to heal itself when you make the right changes to its environment.

PATRIARCHAL MEDICINE

It is important to realise that the conventional medical world, along with our society, despite making many strides forward, is still riddled with patriarchal values. Take the word hysterectomy, this term is taken from the word 'hyster' referring to the womb which was deemed to be the root of women's hysteria / uncontrolled emotional outbursts. Removing it – 'ectomy' – was seen as a quite acceptable way of 'solving' a woman's unacceptable emotional outbursts. I had one client who had a hysterectomy and post the operation her sex hormone levels were tested to see what they were doing. The male doctor delivering the results said 'It's all right Clare, you are still a woman', yes, I was speechless too.

Take the birth control pill, again we are messing about with our hormone levels despite the knowledge that increasing oestrogen levels in the body can:

- Increase risk for cancer
- Increase risk for blood clots
- Cause anxiety and / or depression
- Cause nutrient deficiencies like B vitamins, iron, magnesium, zinc and vitamin C
- Increase risk for yeast overgrowth / candida

Many women I see cannot tolerate the contraceptive pill with oestrogen in it so they take a progesterone-only one, which causes fewer symptoms, but this is also not without its risks:

- Increase risk for breast cancer
- Increase risk of blood clots
- Increased skin issues including acne
- Joint and muscular pain
- Nervous tremors
- Dizziness

I wonder why the male contraceptive pill is not more popular?

The natural processes of a woman's body – menstruation, childbirth and menopause – are seen as something to be controlled and fixed. Medical intervention is always deemed superior to a more natural and non-toxic approach where we work with the body. A study in 2013 looking at the rates of caesarean section showed that those mothers who were supported by a doula (a non-medically-trained person who guides a woman through the childbirth process) throughout their labour had a 40% lower risk of needing a caesarean.[41] This would save a fortune for our NHS but no, doulas, as they are not medically trained, are generally deemed by the medical profession to be hippy, old world meddlers who bring nothing to the birthing party.

For so many hormone imbalance situations, the conventional medical world tends to give pills with more hormones, in a bid to balance, but as you will see from the above case study, very often the body can do this itself if it is given a bit of a helping hand.

I find the same problem with menopause, this is a natural process that the body goes through and it is being medicalised. With regards to HRT I am not totally against it, for some women it can be literally a life saver, but my concern is the one-size-fits-all approach. If you visit the doctor with menopausal symptoms, they usually run a blood test to see if you have raised FSH (follicle-stimulating hormone). If you do, they will very often offer HRT, but with no further testing they don't know which of your hormones actually needs replacing, if they do at all. So many women take HRT that contains oestrogen and they don't need extra oestrogen. This excess of oestrogen can be dangerous as it is one of the main drivers in oestrogen-sensitive cancers, e.g. breast, ovarian and uterine cancers.

If you are really struggling with your hormones, I would advise that firstly you make dietary changes, support the liver to help it deal with fluctuating hormone levels and make sure that you are eating a diet that keeps your blood sugar levels even.

Eat ground flaxseeds (ground is important as the digestive system does not have the ability to break down the tough husk and so therefore cannot benefit from the wonderful essential fats that are contained within). Take 1–2 tablespoons sprinkled on anything and mixed in, make sure that you have them with a glass of water. These are a great source of phytoestrogens, which are natural plant oestrogens, they can balance your levels whether they are too low or too high.

Ensure you are drinking enough water (includes herbal tea but not normal tea and coffee) – your weight in kgs multiplied by 0.033 will give the quantity in litres that you should have daily. A dehydrated liver will really struggle to detox.

Make sure that you are having a daily bowel movement, it is important to expel any excess hormones that the liver has packaged up.

Eat a more paleo-style diet to keep blood sugar levels from swinging up and down – see FOOD Chapter.

Eat foods with isoflavones: chickpeas, alfalfa, fava beans, red clover tea and kudzu. Soya beans also fall into this category but I find that most soya is genetically modified these days (a whole other story) and many people struggle to digest it. Another issue in the West, where we have products like soya milk and yoghurt: the process that the beans have gone through to turn them into milk and yoghurt is fairly toxic, so if you do want to eat soya have it in the fermented form: tofu, tempeh, miso etc, it also means that the body can digest it more easily.

There is a range of herbal remedies that help to support and balance hormones, e.g.

- Black cohosh
- Alfalfa
- Red clover
- Dong quai
- Wild yam
- Ginseng
- Skullcap
- Agnus castus
- Devil's claw

- Evening primrose oil – make sure that it has at least 12% GLA content

There are many different combinations of these out there and I suggest that you experiment with different ones to see which work the best for you. Take care if you are on other medications as some of the herbs can increase or reduce the effect of drugs. If you look at the Medscape drug interaction checker online it is a useful resource for checking any contraindicated herb / drug reactions.

Most importantly it is vital to look at your stress levels and how healthy your adrenal glands are (see STRESS Chapter). When our ovaries run out of eggs and stop producing these sex hormones, the adrenals are the gland that has to take over producing the sex hormones to maintain a balance. If you are driving your adrenals hard, asking them to produce lots of cortisol and adrenalin, then they will not have the reserves to produce sex hormones as well.

WESTERN ATTITUDES TO MENOPAUSE

Our attitude to the menopause in the Western world has a powerful and detrimental effect on the female psyche. Generally, it is viewed with dread, a sign that we are getting older, everything is going to start drying up and that our fertile days are over. For many it is not something that women feel comfortable talking about or admitting to. However, in indigenous societies the menopause is anticipated with more enthusiasm, it is seen as a coming of age – when a woman achieves more status in the community, a time of transformation for body, mind and spirit. This is a time when the focus can be more on ourselves, there is increased liberation from the days of looking after everyone else and putting our needs on the back burner. I am not saying that those days are completely over, as women we are usually all typecast into the role of looking after people, but at least our children don't tend to need us quite so much. It is a time where we have the space for pursuing our unexplored passions and spiritual growth. Personally, I am planning on having a menopause party when the time comes. I have forewarned my children and it will give me a licence to be even more embarrassing.

A BIT FOR THE BOYS

Male hormone balance is a topic that has been hugely neglected, I think partly because women's health is generally much more medicalised and also because men do not generally visit the doctor unless their body is really shouting at them. Men's hormone balance is equally affected by our environment. Besides the issue of too much oestrogen, the most common complaint is low testosterone. Signs of low testosterone are:

- Loss of libido
- Lower sperm count and infertility
- Decreased body hair
- Increased fat around the middle
- Increased breast tissue
- Decreased muscle mass and strength
- Low red blood cells – anaemia
- Decreased bone density
- Increased risk for cardiovascular disease[42]
- Increased fatigue
- Insomnia[43]
- Depression

Low testosterone can be caused by:

- Obesity, especially abdominal obesity as the fat cells convert testosterone to oestrogen.
- Stress – requires the body to make excess amounts of

cortisol which lowers testosterone levels.

- Exposure to external chemical forms of oestrogen
- Taking excessive amounts of exercise
- Medications like opioid painkillers or steroids

If you are experiencing some of the above symptoms, it is worth cleaning up your diet, losing visceral (round the middle) fat if you need to and addressing stress levels. If you are then still struggling ask your doctor for your testosterone levels to be measured. Boosting your testosterone levels if they are too low can make a huge difference to how you feel.

Our hormonal balance, like so many mechanisms in the body, is finely tuned and hugely sensitive to our multi-faceted environment. Many simple changes as in Helen's case can be quite literally life-changing. Sometimes it may be completely necessary to put in some additional bio-identical hormones, but please get your hormone levels checked before you go down this path so that your body is getting what it needs and not a one-size-fits-all protocol.

6

THE GUT

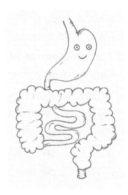

The gut is the most phenomenal invention, and it does far more than just digest our food. It is a fully functioning organ, independent of the brain, with its own enteric nervous system. If you cut the vagus nerve which runs from the brain to the gut, the gut will continue to function perfectly happily without any input from the brain.

The following are some top gut facts
The gut scans our environment by sampling the food that we ingest and feeds messages back to the brain. Research into the vagus nerve has shown that 90% of the information that travels along it goes in the direction of gut to brain.

80% of our immune system is based in the gut.

The bacteria in our gut, often called our gut microbiome, can help to train the immune system to show tolerance –

we are being bombarded constantly by external factors that have the ability to trigger an immune response. People who have hay fever have lost the ability to show tolerance to any of the pollens and dust etc that are flying around in the atmosphere.

Our gut bacteria can dictate what we want to eat. If you have lots of sugar-loving yeast and bacteria living in your gut, they will drive you to eat just that.

We produce most of our brain neurotransmitters in the gut; not only are they produced here but the gut also contains countless receptors for these chemical messengers, serotonin alone has seven different types of receptor – this is why you often feel strong emotions in your gut as well as your brain. There are in fact receptors to these neurotransmitters on every cell, therefore emotions are really felt throughout the entire body, not just in the brain. These chemical messengers, put very simply, include serotonin our happy hormone, dopamine the motivation hormone, GABA the calming down hormone and norepinephrine, which gives a general sense of wellbeing. All of our emotions are a combination of different levels of these neurotransmitters; if gut function is imbalanced it can profoundly affect our mood and behaviour.

Our gut lining is only 1 cell thick (very easy to damage) and the entire lining replaces itself every 4 days.

In 400 bc Hippocrates claimed that:

'All disease begins in the gut.'

He was way ahead of his time – he had no clever diagnostic machines and blood tests to work with, but he did observe and listen to people's bodies. All diseases involve an inflammatory response – this is the immune system's reaction to any form of insult, be it:

infection – bacterial, viral, fungal

trauma – physical or emotional

nutritional deficiencies

The gut is essentially the largest surface area of the body that is exposed to the outside world, so it makes sense for the majority of our immune system to be based just under the surface of the gut wall to intercept any intruders. We ingest 'foods' from our outside environment along with all the 'non-foods' – pesticides, herbicides, medication, in particular antibiotics, food colourings, flavour enhancers, chemical sweeteners etc, and it ends up in the interior of our bodies. The top layer of the gut wall is very delicate and thin, it needs to be that way so that we can absorb food through it, but the downside is that it is very easily damaged. The damage can arise from:

- Alcohol
- Sugar
- Gluten and other grains
- Parasites, yeasts and pathogenic bacteria
- Medication – antibiotics, acid reflux meds, contraceptive pill, NSAIDS (aspirin, ibuprofen, paracetamol)
- Chemotherapy
- Stress

Alcohol – interferes with anti-inflammatory hormones that protect the gut wall, it also interferes with the absorption of nutrients that maintain health.

Sugar – feeds pathogenic bacteria and yeasts, which in turn damage the gut wall. The yeasts in particular can grow through the gut wall and open up the tight junctions between the cells, causing something called leaky gut. Leaky gut can wreak havoc because it means that there is no longer a barrier between anything you ingest – nutrients or toxins – and the bloodstream. When things that should be kept in the gut start leaking through into the interior of the body it upsets the immune system, which then has to be on constant alert. Highly reactive immune systems increase levels of inflammation and can develop into autoimmune situations.

Gluten and other grains – this is a controversial one; we have been eating gluten for centuries, why is it now causing such a problem? The trouble is that the wheat that is grown now has a much higher gluten content. Everyone wants those big puffed-up squidgy loaves, but in order to get that there needs to be a high gluten content. Gluten is like the glue that holds the loaf together as it fills with air from the fermenting yeast. I see copious numbers of clients regain their health when they stop eating gluten. If their gut is really damaged, they need to cut out other grains as well because the immune system that has already developed antibodies to the gluten can cross-react to other grains. In my experience gluten is an important contributing factor to autoimmunity.

Parasites, yeasts and pathogenic bacteria – to put it into perspective, for every one cell in our body we have ten bacteria / microbes in our gut. We are talking about a tube from mouth to anus that is teeming with life, and if this metropolis of bugs is out of balance with the bad guys running the show it can have a profound effect on overall health. We don't have to go on exotic holidays to pick up parasites etc, we have plenty living on our doorstep – if we have a robust gut and a fully functioning immune system these pathogens will not be able to take up residence in any number to cause us harm. However, if our good gut bacteria levels are on the low side then the pathogenic bacteria, yeasts or parasites will dig in and set up home. They will thrive on poorly digested food, sugar and refined carbohydrates, they will produce toxins that damage the gut wall and make it leaky or even burrow right through the gut wall and into the bloodstream. Once in the bloodstream the world is their oyster and they can travel all over the body wreaking havoc wherever they choose. If you get the chance to have some live blood analysis you can see these bugs that are inhabiting your body under the microscope. It can be a little alarming.

Antibiotics – these kill indiscriminately, so that both the good and bad bacteria suffer – often people find that after antibiotics they get some form of fungal infection like thrush; this is because antibiotics, by killing off the good bacteria, leave a bit of a vacuum in the gut, now it is warm and wet in there and yeasts will take advantage of the lack of competition. In many other countries if you are prescribed antibiotics you will automatically be given probiotics to take after your course. Even the NHS website says there is evidence that probiotics can help reduce antibiotic-associated diarrhoea and the risk of Clostridium Difficile infection, so why are probiotics not being provided automatically by the health service?

Perhaps something to do with the fact that probiotics are a naturally occurring phenomena and can't be patented.

Acid Reflux medication – it is estimated that 20% of the adult population endure acid reflux symptoms. In my experience with clients, the figure is much higher. Again, suppressing acid is a sticking-plaster approach and once you are on the medication it is hard to get off it because many people experience rebound symptoms. The most common reason why we get acid reflux symptoms in the first place is because our acid levels are too low – yes I said low. Let me explain, acid in the stomach has two main jobs, firstly to break down our food and secondly to keep the bad bacteria levels under control. Acid production in the stomach is quite hard work for the body, it is pH2, that is nearly the pH of battery acid which can melt steel. As we get older and the environment takes its toll on our bodies, our acid production levels can fall. This means that we then do not digest our food properly and also don't keep the levels of bad bacteria under control. Picture the scenario – you have just eaten a nice big burger in a bun (protein is the hardest food to break down) and your digestive system has not produced enough acid to deal with the meat or the bread, which gets partially broken down. This partially broken down food eventually leaves the stomach – if you don't have enough stomach acid, food hangs around in the stomach, clients often describe it as food sitting like a stone just under the ribcage. This food goes into the small intestine where there is some bacteria but should not be too many (some people can get SIBO, which is Small Intestinal Bacterial Overgrowth, causing all sorts of digestive symptoms – you can test for this). The food then moves into the large intestine where there are lots of bacteria, a mixture of good and bad. The less helpful bacteria thrive more on the meat and grains and they tuck in by fermenting the food to help break it down. The problem with the fermentation is that it creates gas (bloating, belching, flatulence etc) and the pressure from this gas backs up the digestive tract and creates pressure in the stomach which can cause a bit of the acid to leak up into the oesophagus. The oesophagus is the tube running from the mouth to the top of the stomach. In the stomach there is a very thick mucus lining to protect the stomach wall from the acid but as soon as it leaks up into the oesophagus there is no protection from the acid, even acid fumes can cause that burning sensation and eventually lead to cell damage. Other symptoms of acid leaking up from the stomach are:

- Chest pain
- Hoarse, sore throat
- Cough
- Asthma-type symptoms
- Nausea
- Difficulty swallowing
- Excess saliva

Long-term acid reflux can cause so much damage in the oesophagus that the cells can become cancerous, so it is really important that this issue is not ignored. However, usually what patients are not told is that acid suppression with medication often leads to nutrient deficiencies – if we suppress our levels of acid, we are not able to break the food down properly. Long term this can lead to many chronic conditions like osteoporosis,[44] kidney disease[45] and dementia.[46] In order to help our acid reflux it is important to address any gut bacterial imbalance and improve our digestion of food.

IMPROVING OUR DIGESTION OF FOOD

It is all very well eating a perfect diet but if we are not breaking the food down properly and absorbing it then we won't benefit from our virtuous eating.

Allow the cephalic response to kick in

The cephalic response is the production of stomach acid and digestive enzymes that are triggered by sight, smell, thought or taste of food. This response is not given much of a chance to work when we grab something from the fridge and rush around doing jobs whilst eating it.

Try to:

Sit down.

Take 60 seconds to look at your food – start digesting it with your eyes, and smell it. All of these actions give your body time to prepare, getting the stomach acid levels up and producing the digestive enzymes.

Chew – our stomach does not have teeth and the more time the food spends in the mouth the more time the digestive enzymes in the mouth have to do their job.

Concentrate on your eating, try not to multitask when eating – I used to find myself sitting there with the radio on, a magazine in front of me and I was also opening and reading my post – this is not conducive to good digestion. I also had a learnt mechanism for fast eating from school, you did not want to be the last one at the table eating with everyone staring at you. Fast eating is still my default and I have to make a conscious effort to slow down.

Sometimes if the body is tired and under-functioning, concentrating on our eating and slowing it down is just not enough. I would suggest that you try taking some digestive enzymes with your food, which will help you to break it down. Make sure that the supplement enzymes that you take contain:

Protease – to digest protein

Lipase – to digest fat

Amylase – to digest the carbohydrate

It can be helpful to take a teaspoon of apple cider vinegar in half a glass of water with your food to improve the pH in your stomach, although if you are getting acid reflux I would NOT recommend this approach until things have calmed down.

Back to my list of gut damaging things.

Contraceptive pill – oestrogen makes the gut more leaky,[47] and its use has been linked to a higher risk of Crohn's disease.[48] Most contraceptive pills increase the level of oestrogen, which makes the body think that it is pregnant so it doesn't release any more eggs. Extra oestrogen encourages the growth of candida, a yeast that can wreak havoc – I speak from personal experience, by the time I started to address my health I had had candida overgrowth for a couple of decades and as a result was a complete sugar junky because that was what the candida wanted to feed upon. Candida does not just have to stay in the gut – it likes anywhere that is warm and wet. It can travel anywhere in the body and contribute to any of the symptoms below. As you will see the symptoms are hugely diverse.

Possible signs of candida overgrowth
Digestive issues – bloating / flatulence / belching – the yeast likes to ferment what it is feeding upon and this produces gas.

Craving for the sweet stuff – the yeast needs to be fed.

Bad breath – candida produces lots of toxins, which can overload the liver so the liver in desperation will throw toxins out on the breath.

White coating on your tongue – this is the yeast.

Hormone imbalance – the yeast can unpackage oestrogen in the gut, which has already been detoxed by the liver. This oestrogen is then reabsorbed back into the system.

Joint pain – the liver can deposit excess toxins in the joints, causing inflammation.

Chronic sinus issues – the yeast can take up residence in the nasal passages, causing inflammation and excess mucus; a constant frog in the throat can be due to the same thing.

Poor functioning immune system – if the immune system is spending a lot of time trying to get rid of the candida it will not be concentrating on defending the body from other infections so bacterial and viral infections are much more likely and there is an increased risk of cancer.

Low energy – candida runs your system down by over-working the immune system and the liver with excess toxins.

Foggy brain – the excess toxins clog up the brain making it slow and sludgy.

These symptoms can be seen in so many chronic disorders,

it is not always candida that is the culprit; however, if you have vaginal thrush, fungal toenails, athlete's foot or a coated tongue I would suspect that candida / yeast overgrowth is almost certainly part of the picture.

NSAIDS – non-steroidal anti-inflammatory drugs prevent the gut wall from protecting itself from acid in the gut. This in turn damages the cells and makes the gut wall more leaky.[49] This research was done as far back as 1987, so why are we still being prescribed these drugs so regularly?

STRESS

The fight / flight reaction puts digestive function on the back burner, less stomach acid and less digestive enzymes, which can lead to a bacterial imbalance and leaky gut. In addition, stress also makes the gut more permeable so that it is easier to absorb nutrients. When we are in a life-threatening situation it is important that we absorb nutrients very easily so the gut becomes more permeable. The problem is that permanent stress leads to a permanently more permeable gut, this allows things across the gut wall that would not be allowed in under calm circumstances.

Long-term stress can reduce the blood supply to the gut which means that it reduces production of something called Secretory IgA – SIgA's main job is to protect mucosal linings, e.g. the huge surface area that extends from mouth to anus. If the mucosal lining becomes damaged it leads to leakiness and inflammation.

A damaged gut wall leaks food proteins or toxic chemicals from the gut into the bloodstream where it sets off an immune reaction. The immune system recognises that these substances are not supposed to be where they are and so it creates antibodies to the food proteins.

ARISE THE FOOD INTOLERANCE

An issue that has only reared its head in the last 30 years.

The diet eaten now in the West is very limited, people are eating the same foods day in and day out, which means that the antibodies that the immune system is producing against these foods reach high levels. In Japan where longevity is superior to the West they are advised to try to eat 30 different foods a day – I have tried it and its quite a challenge, they have lots of small portions of fermented vegetables which means that they consume a much wider and better balanced range of nutrients on a daily basis.

Just for the record, I am not a fan of food intolerance testing. I get many clients coming to me who have had allergy testing done and they have a whole raft of foods that they are reacting to. It is also a rather expensive test to have done. If we have a leaky gut and get a test done, the results can be quite alarming as our body may have started to produce antibodies to many of the foods that we are currently eating. Clients are quite understandably desperate – 'What on earth can I eat?' – but if you do manage to remove all of these foods from your diet you are not actually resolving the problem; symptoms may subside but then you are left with an incredibly restricted diet forever, as you have not fixed the underlying reason why the gut became leaky in the first place. If we can fix this, then we should be able tolerate most of the foods we were reacting to. I will just say that if you are obviously reacting to a certain food then it would be wise to cut it out whilst you are healing the gut. My basic premise is that if we were not reacting to these foods when we were born then it should be possible to get the body back to its factory default setting.

Whilst you are trying to sort out the gut, I recommend removing some of the most regularly offending foods that may be producing symptoms, e.g. gluten and dairy. Trying to work out which foods you are reacting to is often a minefield because you have to remember that the body is always trying to maintain the status quo. Sometimes you may eat a piece of bread and not get symptoms but if you have had a stressed day at work and haven't slept the night before and have perhaps had a few drinks and eaten lots of sugar, then the body burden is too great to maintain the status quo and you are more likely to get symptoms. If clients really want to understand what they are reacting to I tend to put them on an elimination diet. There are various levels of this; if you have a fairly good idea about what you are reacting to then be strict about cutting that food out, if you haven't a clue then try a strict elimination diet – no grains, no dairy, no eggs, no nuts, no soy, no alcohol, no nightshades, no shellfish or fish – yes hideous, basically you are eating vegetables and a bit of good-quality organic protein, ideally grass-fed meat, for three weeks. You can then introduce foods one at a time and watch for symptoms, I also recommend doing the pulse test.

Pulse test

To measure your pulse, place the index and middle finger (not the thumb as it has its own pulse) over the underside of the opposite wrist, below the base of the thumb. Press firmly with flat fingers until you feel the pulse in the radial artery. Record how many beats per minute you get – this is your pulse rate.

Please note that smoking may affect results. The pulse test is done by taking your pulse several times for a couple of days to get to know what your average pulse rate at rest is, keep a record of this.

To test – ensure that the food that you are testing has not been ingested at all for three weeks prior to taking the test.

Take your pulse seated before the meal and prior to ingesting any food or drink and record it.

After consuming the test food (don't go mad with the quantity but make sure it is enough to get a reaction, e.g. 1 slice of bread etc) take your pulse 5, 10, 20, 30 and 60 minutes after the food.

An increase in pulse rate of more than 10 would indicate that the food is provoking a reaction in the body.

Food intolerances can be reversed, but to do this you need to heal up the gut. Firstly, it is important to ensure that there is nothing living in the gut that is damaging the gut wall. I am a huge fan of stool tests, unfortunately in my experience the general stool tests that are available on the NHS are wholly inadequate. If you have one of the big bad guys like Giardia, C Difficile or Salmonella, it will be picked up, however, there are numerous other bacteria we can harbour in our guts which can cause long-term problems and which will not be tested for with an NHS test. These bacteria may not give dramatic symptoms, but they often give digestive ones that rumble on or have a more slow, insidious effect on overall health – joint / muscle pain, low energy levels, brain fog, migraines, skin problems, depression etc. In fact, when you look at the way these bacteria / parasites can burrow through the wall of the gut and get access to the bloodstream and then travel around the body, they can cause any type of symptom that you choose to name. If you have an infection then this is when you need professional help from somebody who understands the nature of these parasites and bacteria. These bacteria can be very challenging to get rid of but I assure you it is well worth it. Secondly, once you have managed to eradicate the bad guys or reduce their levels so that they are not causing symptoms, it is important to ensure that you are eating a diet that feeds and encourages the growth of the good bacteria.

HEALING THE GUT WALL

A priority is to get your gut bacteria balanced, you can eat lots of gut healing things but if the gut flora contains too many of the bad guys then they will maintain the leakiness of your gut.

Bad bacteria thrives on sugar / refined carbohydrates.

Good bacteria likes to eat prebiotic foods e.g. onions, leeks, garlic, asparagus, chicory, Jerusalem artichoke, broccoli, Brussels sprouts, cabbage, cauliflower, kale, almonds, peas, pistachios, flax, bananas, sweet potato, radish and dandelion leaves (Peter Rabbit had excellent gut bacteria).

Additionally, in order to boost the levels of and increase the diversity of good bacteria species, eat and drink more fermented foods like:

- Sauerkraut
- Kimchi
- Kefir
- Kombucha
- Miso

It is quite easy to make your own fermented foods, in the past I have made sauerkraut and kefir (and fermented fish, the subject of which we will gloss over quickly, suffice to say it was not a success and if I expect to remain in the family home I will not be trying it again). I am now at a kombucha phase (fermented green tea) with large kilner jars in the kitchen with weird jellyfish-like creatures. The jellyfish / SCOBY (Symbiotic Culture of Bacteria and Yeast, which is what you need to be able to ferment the green tea) produces a baby about every 6 weeks which is a little stressful for me as I hate the idea of throwing babies away and try to get them adopted by family and friends at every opportunity – beware, if you come to visit you might leave with more than you bargained for. Kombucha tastes a bit like vinegary apple juice, really not bad and even my children will drink it. If time is short, you can buy these products – see RESOURCES.

There are lots of good probiotic supplements out there but there are also some which are a waste of money. If it is possible, I prefer to balance the gut with food, however sometimes if there is a real imbalance you may have to take supplements as well to help keep the good bacteria in charge. If this approach does not bring relief, I recommend professional help and getting a comprehensive stool analysis done so that you know what you are working with.

GUT BACTERIA AND RED MEAT CONSUMPTION

The wrong bacteria can change normal healthy food into a toxic substance. If the bad ones are running the show, then they can convert the choline in red meat into something called trimethylamine N-oxide (TMAO).[50] TMAO can increase the amount of atherosclerosis (build-up of fatty material on blood vessel walls) which leads to heart disease. So, while the saturated fat content of red meat has always been blamed for causing heart disease it is actually an imbalance in gut bacteria that is the culprit. In order to protect ourselves against heart attacks it is helpful to eat a diet high in fibre and prebiotic foods to ensure that our good bacteria are well fed and keep the bad bacteria under control.[51]

The benefits of bone broth

I wish there was a more attractive name. Bone broth conjures up for me a bit of a witches' cauldron moment 'eye of newt and toe of frog', but I can assure you it is delicious and is incredibly simple to make. I tend to make it from a whole chicken but you can use any other bones and meat. As you are extracting all the goodness from these bones etc I would advise that you try to get organic bones, so that you are not also extracting toxins into your bone broth. The benefit of consuming bone broth is that the minerals like magnesium, calcium, phosphorus, silicon and sulphur are pulled out of the bones and are easily digested in the gut. Additionally, gelatin, which comes from the cartilage and general icky bits around the bone (and gives your bone broth that jiggly / jelly-like texture when it has been in the fridge) contains proteins that help to heal up the gut wall. One of the proteins, glycine, also helps to stimulate digestion. This is a very easy food to digest so if you have a really malfunctioning digestive system, I cannot recommend it highly enough for getting good nutrition that won't tax your digestion. Bone broth is a large part of the Gut and Psychology Syndrome Diet that has such wonderful results with helping autistic and ADHD children.

Basic recipe

1 whole organic chicken or other bones and meat – the more gristly bits the better.

Any vegetables (not potato) or herbs you like but I would always include garlic and onions if your gut will tolerate them.

A pinch of Himalayan rock salt and some black pepper – not compulsory but adds to the flavour.

1 tablespoon of apple cider vinegar – this makes the liquid very slightly acid which helps to pull out the alkalising minerals from the bones.

Put all ingredients in a large stainless-steel pot and fill up with filtered water. Bring to the boil and then simmer with the lid on for at least 6 hours, the longer you can simmer it the more nutrients will be released from the bones. I usually cook it for up to 24 hours. If you have an Aga / Everhot type cooker I put it in a lower oven at 80 degrees overnight.

Strain off the liquid and drink – it will keep in the fridge for up to a week but if you have excess it freezes well (ideally in a glass container). All the meat from the chicken etc can be picked off and used in other recipes or you can add some of it back to the broth for a more substantial meal. If you have cooked it for a long time the bones will be soft and you can crush them up and feed them to dogs / cats if you have them.

If all this sounds like too much faff you can buy good-quality organic broth from grass-fed animals – see RESOURCES.

GUT SYMPTOMS THAT SHOULD NOT BE IGNORED

Acid reflux / heartburn

Diarrhoea – long term it will lead to nutritional deficiencies as the transit time is too quick for your body to break down and absorb nutrients.

Gas – belching, bloating, flatulence – the pathogenic bacteria are having a feeding frenzy which creates gas. I am not talking about a little bit of windy wind when you have eaten beans, it is more about large quantities of often 'clear the room' kind of flatulence.

Nausea – often comes from the liver and can be a sign of toxicity.

Intestinal pain or spasms – pain can come from all sorts of causes – it is advisable to investigate.

Constipation – this is a hugely underestimated problem. Just so that we are clear you should be having a bowel movement at least once every day, ideally after every meal. I asked one of my clients about his bowel movements and he said 'Oh they're normal'; I asked him how often he moved his bowels and he said 'Once a week!' I can assure you this is anything but normal, this chap had many chronic issues and most of them stemmed from toxicity.

A very important job that the lower bowel performs is water reabsorption because when your food arrives in the large bowel it will be liquid and the body does not want to lose all of that water. If your waste is sitting in the lower bowel for longer than it should, more and more water gets reabsorbed until you end up with rabbit droppings. By the way, we are aiming for a daily smooth sausage in case you were wondering – number 4 on the chart below. The problem is that along with the extra water that gets reabsorbed, you also reabsorb lots of toxins from the stool that have been packaged up by the liver to be sent out of the body. These toxins then re-enter the bloodstream and are carried back to the liver to be dealt with once again. The detoxing mechanism in the liver takes a lot of energy so can make you feel tired if the liver is being overworked, which generally in our 21st-century world it is.

It is a good idea to get into the habit of glancing at your stools on a regular basis – apologies for the graphic display but I find this chart invaluable for clients who feel uncomfortable about delving into details.

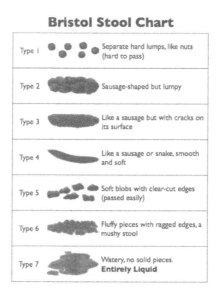

Bristol Stool Chart

Type 1	Separate hard lumps, like nuts (hard to pass)
Type 2	Sausage-shaped but lumpy
Type 3	Like a sausage but with cracks on its surface
Type 4	Like a sausage or snake, smooth and soft
Type 5	Soft blobs with clear-cut edges (passed easily)
Type 6	Fluffy pieces with ragged edges, a mushy stool
Type 7	Watery, no solid pieces. **Entirely Liquid**

Good bacteria can manufacture vitamins
Such as B vitamins, vital for energy production, and vitamin K for blood clotting and bone health. Make sure if you are taking supplements to support bone health they include vitamin K2. Everyone gets carried away with the idea that calcium is the most important and only bone nutrient – there are many others including magnesium, boron, phosphorus, vitamin D, vitamin C, zinc and good-quality protein.

The importance of birth for the gut bacteria

When we are in the uterus our digestive tract is completely sterile, no bacteria in sight. When we travel down the birth canal, if our mother has good levels of beneficial bacteria, we will pick up that bacteria which will start to populate our own digestive tract. This system relies on our mothers having good levels of bacteria, but often now this is not the case for the many reasons above. There are also many more babies being born by caesarean section (approximately 1 in 4 in the UK); this means that the baby will pick up bacteria from the first thing that it comes into contact with, the surgeon's or nurse's hands or cloth that is used to wipe the baby before it is handed to the mother. My eldest son was trying to arrive into the world backwards (bless him) and I ended up with an emergency caesarean; needless to say he had gut problems in early life. If only I had known this information then. Now with caesarean births some forward-thinking midwives are swabbing the birth canal and wiping the baby over with this swab to ensure that they start life with the right bacteria. It is then helpful if that baby is breastfed as there will be continued transfer of beneficial bacteria to the child. I would always recommend that pregnant and breast-feeding mothers ensure that they are ingesting good bacteria either with a variety of probiotics or fermented foods so they can be passing on the best possible bacteria to their babies and giving them the greatest start in life.

As a final point, whilst we are on the subject of micro-biomes, recent research is showing that different areas of the body have their own microbiome which can greatly impact the health of that organ, e.g. the breast has its own microbiome and so does the brain. Keeping the balance of these different microbiomes is key to long-term health and wellbeing.

7

SLUDGE – TOXICITY

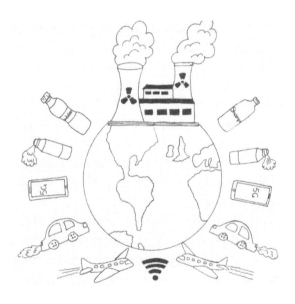

'Concern for man himself and his fate must always form the chief interest of all technical endeavours … in order that the creations of our minds shall be a blessing and not a curse to mankind.'   — Einstein

Apologies, there is no way of softening the blow – our 21st-century environment is very toxic to the human body, unless you live at the top of Alaska (and even that is now no guarantee). Wherever we go, we are surrounded by toxins, and everybody has differing abilities to detox. If you have chronic disease and are not getting the results that you want, I suggest that you look at your toxic exposure. Individual genetic makeups can mean that mutations prevent a smooth flow of the detox pathways in the liver. You can run a genetic test but they are costly and you will need a functional medicine practitioner to help you decipher them. I would start with the guidance in this chapter first, this can go a long way to support your liver and get you a cleaner body. When genes get overwhelmed with toxins they can act as if they are mutated even if they are not.

So many of the chemicals in our environment are tested and deemed safe, but usually with these tests they are a single exposure of that individual chemical. This does not take into account a lifetime's drip-feed exposure that we have to a whole myriad of chemicals that the body does not recognise. A single exposure is unlikely to make you keel over, but the accumulation over time can create a huge burden.

Let me run you through an average day of a person (a hermaphrodite). I have underlined the problem areas and will expand on them below.

You wake up in your lovely cosy <u>bed</u> and check your <u>phone</u>, which has been beside you monitoring your sleep or just acting as an alarm clock. You climb out of bed, stumble to the shower where you wash with <u>soap</u>, <u>shampoo</u>, <u>conditioner</u>, <u>body scrub</u> etc. You then brush your teeth with <u>toothpaste</u> making sure you scrub well around those <u>mercury fillings</u>, then rinse with <u>mouthwash</u>, shave, slap on the <u>aftershave</u>, don't forget to take your <u>contraceptive pill</u>, use <u>antiperspirant</u>. Dress in those freshly <u>laundered</u> and <u>fragranced</u> clothes, apply <u>moisturiser</u>, <u>lip balm</u>, <u>make-up</u>, <u>hairspray</u>, <u>hair gel</u>. And this is all within an hour of getting up.

Breakfast – non-organic <u>cereal / bread</u>, wash dishes without <u>gloves</u>, <u>don't rinse</u> the bubbles off the plates and leave to dry. Out the door – transport to work in <u>brand new car</u>, <u>bike</u>, <u>train</u>, <u>plane</u> into the <u>city / town</u>. Into work surrounded by computers, fire retardants, where they have just smartened up the office with a new paint job, air con and then breathe in or have exposure for the next 8 hours to chemicals at work. At lunchtime you eat your salami / ham sandwich that has been encased in plastic, sat by a colleague who is wearing overpowering perfume, outside in the park with sunscreen on, you then return to the office via the shop to get some tampons with a bit of a headache and take a paracetamol. Meeting in the afternoon in another building, with fresh and different chemicals – commute home, but on the way go to a mammogram appointment, collect clothes from the dry cleaners, get your nails done, have a spray tan and hair appointment to get your hair coloured (big weekend coming up). Then home to sink into that new sofa which has been treated with fire retardant and will be off-gassing for the next two years even though you can't smell anything. Feeling a bit dehydrated so drink lots of unfiltered water, and then consume dinner – tuna fried in a non-stick pan, non-organic vegetables roasted in a pan on a layer of aluminium foil to save on washing up and some delicious-looking strawberries fresh from Peru and then watch the evening news and fall into bed after toothpaste, soap, moisturiser etc.

Before I go through the toxins in more detail, I think it might be helpful to tell you about an experiment that I did on my youngest son when he was 3 (I don't usually experiment on my children apart from giving them weird food, but he is now a strapping 19-year-old so survived to tell the tale). I crushed up some garlic, put it on the bottom of his foot, wrapped his foot up and waited – within 30 minutes his breath started to smell. I was blown away and rather concerned, all that bubble bath that I had been putting in their baths etc, I was poisoning my children. Anything that we put on our skin gets absorbed into the bloodstream.

In addition, anything you inhale also gets into the body, it goes into the lungs and gets absorbed into the bloodstream, which then circulates around. Perfumed washing powders and cleaning products, scents, aftershaves, air fresheners, smell of new car, carpets, curtains etc. Some can even trigger a headache in the sensitive individual – if you are one of those people try to listen to your body rather than taking a paracetamol.

Below is a more detailed list of the environmental toxins that an average person is exposed to. In the RESOURCES section there are many alternative non-toxic products.

Bed – mattress
I also want to put into this category sofas, carpets and curtains, which unless you haven't changed anything for decades will have been treated with fire retardant. One of the most popular ones is TDCPP (1,3-dichloro-2-propyl phosphate), which has been found to affect cell growth and be neurotoxic (toxic to the nervous system and the brain) which is most concerning as this retardant until the 1970s was used in the fabric of children's pyjamas – it was banned in clothing as a possible carcinogen so why is it deemed safe to put into mattresses, sofas, carpets and curtains?

Toxic Hot Seat is a documentary on this topic explaining the toxicity of fire retardants, and also that they do not always make objects more fire resistant.

Phone
Into this category also come computers, laptops, iPads, fitness bands, radiation from power lines and all the electrical objects that surround us on a daily basis that are not hardwired in. All of the above give off electromagnetic radiation (EMR) / radio frequency radiation (RFR) which affects us because most of the chemical reactions in the human body rely on an electrical charge. In 1983 the first mobile phones went on sale in the US, now more people have

mobile phones than people who own a loo: this is an enormous change for the body to cope with. We are living in a toxic soup of EMR and it is only going to get worse. The following is an extract from research into radio frequency radiation (RFR).[52]

> A broad range of adverse human health effects associated with RFR (radio frequency radiation) have been reported … three large-scale carcinogenicity studies in rodents exposed to levels of RFR that mimic lifetime human exposures have shown significantly increased rates of Schwannomas and malignant gliomas [e.g. cancer] as well as chromosomal DNA damage. Of particular concern are the effects of RFR exposure on the developing brain in children. Compared with an adult male, a cell phone held against the head of a child exposes deeper brain structures to greater radiation doses per unit volume, and the young, thin skull's bone marrow absorbs a roughly 10-fold higher local dose. Experimental and observational studies also suggest that men who keep cell phones in their trouser pockets have significantly lower sperm counts and significantly impaired sperm motility and morphology, including mitochondrial DNA damage.

It is important with research to ascertain who is carrying it out, and a large proportion is at the behest of the industry themselves, who are keen for their product to come out smelling of roses, no matter what harm it might be doing to the individual. Despite the mixed results about the dangers of EMR or EMF (electromagnetic frequency) I have clients (including myself) who are sensitive to it: the official name for this is EHS Electromagnetic Hypersensitivity, a recognised condition. It tends to be more obvious in those with Chronic Fatigue type symptoms, where the body's levels of resilience are lower. It is often difficult to pinpoint that EMR is the culprit, as symptoms can be so varied. These can be:

A warm tingling or burning sensation or pain on the face / ear or hand where you have been holding the phone

A tingling or prickling sensation in other parts of the body

Issues with mucous membranes – either too dry or swelling

Brain fog, including low concentration, loss of memory and dizziness

Headaches

Nausea

Feeling of general malaise that never develops into anything

Very rapid heartbeat / palpitations

Depression

Unexplained fear / anxiety

Fatigue

Disrupted sleep

EMR exposure has been linked to increased risk for:

Low sperm count and fertility issues

Neurodegenerative diseases

Type 2 diabetes

Type 1 diabetes

Cardiovascular disease

Cancer

ADHD

HOW EXACTLY DOES EMR AFFECT THE BODY

All cells in your body are sensitive to EMR – just look up the effect of EMR on ants on YouTube and you will see what happens to them with an incoming call. Cells are far smaller and more vulnerable than ants. Martin Pall, who wrote *Explaining Unexplained Illnesses* discovered that EMR adversely affects the voltage-gated calcium channels in the cell – these are channels in the cell membrane that control how much calcium is allowed into the cell and they are powered by low levels of electricity. If these channels are exposed to EMR they remain open so that the cell becomes flooded with calcium. Excessive amounts of calcium in the cell means that the cell gets 'overexcited' so that the cell function speeds up excessively, which can lead to cell death. If the cell doesn't die we have an overactive cell, which will produce different effects depending upon which organ that cell is part of. It could be excessive muscular contraction – this is unlikely to mean that you will get involuntary muscle contraction, but on a more subtle level tight muscles lead to musculoskeletal issues and inflammation. Over-excitation of neurons: worst-case scenario is epilepsy but on a more subtle level could it be contributing to our staggering rise of ADHD-type issues in children – evidence seems to be showing that this is the case.[53] Excessive release of hormones can cause havoc in the body. We are not just talking about the sex hormones here, there are over 60 hormones performing functions that range from dictating how fast your metabolism runs, to how well you sleep, to how fast your gut works, to how many red blood cells you produce.

In a world where our body is already over-stimulated, EMR exposure is just adding fuel to the fire.

Something else that I discovered whilst looking into EMR is that it can make your blood–brain barrier more leaky (increased risk for Parkinson's, dementia and Alzheimer's). In fact, there are various barriers to protect different organs: the gut wall barrier (increased risk for autoimmune diseases), the ocular barrier which protects the eyes (increased risk for cataracts), and the placental barrier which protects the foetus. If these barriers are leaky, they cannot block out the toxins.

EMR effect on children

Children are more sensitive to EMR than adults because their cells have a higher water content so the EMR can penetrate more easily, particularly in the brain where their skull is not so thick. France seems to be leading the way with laws about banning Wi-Fi in nurseries and keeping its use to a minimum in elementary schools. Many public buildings and universities have removed Wi-Fi and all phones must display radiation levels and be sold with headsets. The UK, on the other hand, does not seem to be so forward thinking. The NHS guidelines are as follows, with the first sentence on the mobile phone safety page reading:

'Research suggests it's unlikely that mobile phones or base stations increase the risk of health problems.'

And this is what they had to say with regard to mobile phone use and children:

> If there are any health risks from the use of mobile phones, children might be more vulnerable because their bodies and nervous systems are still developing.
>
> Research carried out to date hasn't supported a link between mobile phone use and childhood cancers such as leukaemia.
>
> However, if you have any concerns, you can lower your child's exposure to radio waves by only allowing them to use mobile phones for essential purposes and keeping calls short.

I'm not sure I am prepared to take the chance on the 'unlikelihood' of there being a risk.

If this is not all depressing enough, the situation will worsen with the introduction of 5G because 5G works on a very different technology to 4G and is 1,000 times more powerful. It is based upon microwave radiation, the very same technology that governments have employed to develop weaponry. If you subject a population to this microwave radiation at a very low dose you can cause neurological problems and increased rates of cancer. When Bristol University trialled 5G in 2017 there was an increase in student suicide rates that year. A link is going to be very hard to prove but somebody should be looking into it. If you want to learn more about this subject, I urge you to watch the film *5G Apocalypse* on YouTube and please sign anything that you can to campaign against it.

If you think EMR may be an issue for you, see advice at the end of this chapter.

Shower
We have a double whammy here, the water and shower curtains – most shower curtains are made from PVC which contain VOCs (volatile organic compounds), these have been found to damage the liver, kidneys and nervous system, also phthalates, which contain hormone-disrupting chemicals, responsible for early breast development in girls and feminisation of baby boys. It is possible to buy shower curtains made from hemp – see RESOURCES.

Water
Our water supply is a hotbed of toxins. Firstly fluoride – some areas in the UK have fluoride added to their water,[54] fluoride being a neurotoxin and a hormone disruptor. Then come all the pesticides, herbicides, heavy metals and chlorine, and finally the really problematic substance oestrogen. Most women on the contraceptive pill (many contraceptive pills contain oestrogen) will be peeing excess oestrogen into our water supply, the water companies know that this is an issue but oestrogen is a difficult and expensive substance to filter out so they are sticking their heads in the sand about it. Until the government brings in some regulation on this, things are unlikely to change and we will all continue to consume excess oestrogen. The filter jugs that sit in your fridge are not effective enough to filter out oestrogen. There are

I Wish My Doctor Had Told Me This

water filter systems that you can get for the whole house, which I advise if you have a chronically ill person, but otherwise it's enough to make sure that the water you are drinking and cooking with is toxin-free. See RESOURCES for under-the-sink reverse osmosis filters: these are the most effective at filtering toxins, especially substances like oestrogen.

Toiletries

Soap, shampoo, conditioner, deodorant, antiperspirant, make-up, face wash, aftershave, moisturiser, mouthwash, toothpaste, hair products ... the list of lotions and potions that we use on our bodies is endless.

Some of the ingredients to look out for in toiletries are:

Parabens – contain oestrogen-mimicking substances linked to breast / prostate cancer.

Fragrance – a blanket term which doesn't actually say what it is – the company could be using anything but generally fragrances have been classed as irritants affecting the immune system.

Pthalates – also used in plastics to increase their flexibility. Pthalates contain hormone-disrupting chemicals.

Triclosan – an antimicrobial chemical known to disrupt thyroid and reproductive hormones, there are also concerns that it is contributing to the development of anti-biotic-resistant bacteria.

Sodium lauryl sulphates – these create foaming products which are irritating to skin, lungs and eyes; in addition, they can combine with other chemicals to form nitrosamines which are known carcinogens.

Formaldehyde – used for preserving dead bodies. Classed as a human carcinogen and harmful to the immune system.

PEGs – skin irritant.

Toluene – derived from petroleum and used as a paint

thinner, linked to autoimmune disease and developmental damage of foetuses.

Aluminium in deodorants and anti-perspirants – aluminium is a toxic metal, particularly to the brain[55] as it promotes the growth of the tau protein, which is a prime factor in the development of Alzheimer's. These products are spread / sprayed all over the underarm where there is a dense network of lymph glands. Once the aluminium is absorbed by the skin the lymph makes it very easy for the aluminium to travel around the body.

Doesn't make for a pretty picture – again as with food, most manufacturers are not interested in our wellbeing: they want to make products that make us look and smell good, but at what cost to our health?

If you are keen on your bath products and want to make your own bath bombs try this recipe below.

You will need:

Bath Bombs
Dry ingredients:
¼ cup food-grade diatomaceous earth
¼ cup Epsom salts
½ cup citric acid
½ cup cornstarch
1 cup baking soda – get the Arm & Hammer variety as this does not contain aluminium
Wet ingredients:
2 tbsp essential oil – use whichever smells you like best
2 tsp olive oil
1 tbsp coconut oil
¾ tbsp water
3–4 drops of organic non-toxic food colouring (optional) see Resources
You will need:

A mixing bowl
A spray bottle
Large ice cube trays

Step 1:
Place food-grade diatomaceous earth, Epsom salts, citric acid, cornstarch, and baking soda in your mixing bowl. Mix these ingredients evenly.

Step 2:
Pour essential oil (whatever scent you choose), olive oil, coconut oil, water, and food colouring in a spray bottle and shake thoroughly. You may need to warm this mixture to ensure that the coconut oil melts.

Step 3:
While stirring, spritz some of the wet mixture into the dry mixture. If you were to add all of the wet mixture at once, the baking soda and citric acid would react. By adding the wet mixture slowly, you prevent this.
The mixture should reach a consistency similar to wet sand (where you can cake it together in your hand). If your mixture is not the right consistency, add a little more food colouring and water to the spray bottle and continue to add the coloured water slowly.

Step 4:
Once the mixture has reached the consistency of wet sand, take some and pack it tightly into your ice cube tray.

Step 5:
Store in a dry place for 12–24 hours. The bath bombs should harden and resemble giant gobstoppers. Remove the bath bombs from the ice cube tray and put in a sealed glass jar to keep them dry.

To use your bath bombs, simply add to your bathwater. They will fizz and spread the essential oils and diatomaceous earth throughout the water.

For a simple moisturiser I use coconut oil at night, it does mean that you clamber into bed a bit shiny and smelling like a Bounty bar, but this is a small price to pay for a cleaner body.

Deodorant versus anti-perspirant
Sweating is one of the body's important detox mechanisms; I would always recommend on a day-to-day basis that people use an aluminium-free deodorant rather than an anti-perspirant, which actually stops your body from sweating. See RESOURCES.

Toothpaste
Most contain fluoride which is a poison – in the US this is the label on all fluoride-containing toothpastes:

'WARNING: Keep out of reach of children under 6 years of age. If you accidentally swallow more than used for brushing, seek professional help or contact a poison control center immediately.'[56]

Because fluoride belongs to the same chemical family as iodine it can also disrupt thyroid function.

Mercury amalgams
Mercury is a known heavy metal – which the dental industry claims to be safe. By placing it in our mouths we then get a slow-drip-feed of a toxin. Heavy metals have the ability to displace zinc in the body and zinc is a key nutrient involved in over 300 enzyme reactions which are critical to tissue growth and repair, wound healing and hormone balance. As an aside, the white fillings can also be toxic, some contain Bisphenol A, which can interfere with thyroid function and

is a known carcinogen. If you are getting white fillings ask your dentist what is contained in the composite they use. Don't be afraid to make a fuss and ask them to source a non-toxic variety. If they won't, find another dentist who will – look up IAOMT.org for biological dentists. I feel the more that we make a fuss as a nation, the more the use of non-toxic dental products will become mainstream.

MY DENTAL STORY

At the age of 16 I got my top two front teeth smashed by a hockey-ball, this was before the days of gum guards. My teeth were fixed but the trauma to that part of my mouth meant that a very slow insidious infection in the gum started, which damaged one of the teeth next to the two front ones. Fast forward 19 years to 2005 and I ended up with a root canal. I had no idea at the time that root canals were the cause of so many chronic health problems. Root canals I understand on the face of it seem like a good idea because you are keeping the original tooth in place but when you think about it, this is a dead tooth and it doesn't make sense to keep dead tissue in the body and not expect it to cause problems. With a root canal, the nerve is removed, leaving a warm wet cavity with no blood supply to fight infection. The infection starts slowly and the body does its best to fight, in fact doing such a good job that it usually does not manifest any pain, so it is difficult to know there is a problem apart from the fact that I felt lousy and had developed fibromyalgia. By 2019 when I went to see a holistic dentist, the infection was so bad that I had to have my three front teeth removed and a bone graft (the infection had eaten away at the bone with a bone loss of size approximately 12mm x 8mm x 5mm) so that they could put some implants in. This has been a rather slow and painful process. After the bone graft, my youngest commented that I could have auditioned for *Planet of the Apes* my face was

so swollen – don't you just love 'em. As I write I am about
to go and get my implants done – this will take a further
three months to heal before I actually get some teeth. If you
have any chronic health problems and you have had a root
canal I suggest that you watch the film *Root Cause* – the
presentation of this film is rather over-dramatic, but it will
give you a clear picture of what root canals are all about and
how much they can affect our health – and if possible find
a biological dentist to help you.

Contraceptive pill
The World Health Organization has classified the combined
(oestrogen and progesterone) pill and HRT (hormone re-
placement therapy) as carcinogenic. The contraception
question is a difficult one. We should think very long and
hard about taking a medication that affects our levels of hormones because they are not without consequence.

Washing powder
Laundry product manufacturers are not required to list all
the ingredients in their products. My suggestion is that you
try to buy environmentally friendly / organic brands (see
RESOURCES) and watch out for the ingredients below.

Benzaldehyde – bleach / perfume, irritant causing cough,
sore throat, redness and pain to eyes and skin.

Ethyl acetate – fabric softener – 4 hours of exposure
to ethyl acetate at concentrations of 16,000ppm was
enough to kill 6 rats – now I am not suggesting that
there are levels this high in your washing powder but it
makes you think.

Nonylphenol ethoxylate – detergent – detected in human breast milk, blood and urine – skin irritant.

Quaternium-15 – detergent – releases formaldehyde, a
carcinogen.

Non-organic food

The chemicals that are used in food production are numerous and varied; to avoid the risk of you falling asleep I won't go into all of them, but one I will mention is glyphosate or Roundup. There has been much in the press about this chemical – the most used agricultural chemical in history. Due to genetically modified crops, it can now be sprayed liberally on to crops without damaging them, but humans are ingesting this chemical at toxic levels. Glyphosate has the effect of damaging the microbiome of the soil (all the beneficial bacteria that help to produce healthy plants and act as a natural weedkiller). Translate this into the human body and it does the same thing, it damages our gut bacteria levels and makes the gut more leaky. Dr Stephanie Seneff has spent many years researching this problem and has uncovered some very damning evidence on the link between glyphosate use and the increase in autism, cancer and inflammatory bowel disease. In 2015 the International Agency for Research on Cancer classified glyphosate as a 'probable carcinogen'.[57] More recently there have been some high profile lawsuits brought against Monsanto (the manufacturers of glyphosate) where juries have found that not only does glyphosate cause cancer but that Monsanto knew about the risks and hid the information from consumers.[58] [59]

The tide is slowly starting to turn but we are talking about dealing with huge corporations, who will protect their product no matter what. We as the consumers need to be effecting change by refusing to consume these products. In addition to what is being put on our growing food, our bodies then have to contend with all of the chemicals that food manufacturers are putting in our foods in a bid to make them cheap, sweet, salty, crispy etc. If you want to delve further into the subject of what ends up in our food, I recommend reading Joanna Blythman's book *Swallow This*. Joanna is an investigative food journalist who has dug up some very disturbing facts about what the food manufacturers put into our food in a bid to make more profits.

Washing up liquid, rinse aid, dishwasher tablets
Unless you diligently rinse all dishes and pans when you are washing up then there will be residues left, which you will end up consuming – we are talking tiny quantities here but over time this all adds to the toxic load. I am extremely bossy when people wash up in my house and ask them 'politely' to rinse everything. I have also swapped my dishwasher tablets to a homemade powder (see recipe below) and the rinse aid to distilled white vinegar. Dishwashers do not rinse the dishes sufficiently and the rinse water contains rinse aid. Using these alternatives means that if you do ingest some it will not be harmful. I am, however, aware of my extreme habits, if you feel that life is too short to make your own dishwasher powder see RESOURCES section.

Chemical-free dishwasher powder
4 cups of baking soda
1 cup of citric acid
1 cup of coarse salt – make sure the salt is very dry before you mix it or it goes into a solid mass
20-25 drops of essential oil – lemon, orange or grapefruit
Mix all together and use a teaspoon in normal loads or tablespoon in extra-dirty loads
Use distilled white vinegar in the rinse aid compartment.

New car
That new car smell – full of plastics, adhesives, heavy metals and sealants that are off-gassing. Many of these substances are recognised as toxic to human health.[60]

If you have a new car – get the windows open as much as you can till the smell subsides – it can be for up to a year.

Diesel / petrol fumes
These have been shown to promote cardiovascular problems, lung disease, cancer and toxicity to the brain. The evidence about petrol fumes that I cite comes from research done in 1913![61] [62] It is a difficult problem to solve but the more the general public are saying this is not acceptable, the faster we will progress. If you exercise / ride a bike in a town or city, I urge you to wear a mask, they take a little getting used to but better than breathing in toxic fumes when you are supposedly doing something beneficial for the body.

Sick building syndrome
The office environment is found to be particularly bad in open plan offices. This is a recognised problem by the NHS that can produce a range of symptoms, thought to be caused by:
- Poor ventilation
- Fluctuations in temperature
- Inhaled dust, fungal / mould spores, carpet fibres
- Air conditioning
- Electromagnetic radiation
- Poor lighting causing glare from screens
- Fumes from cleaning products, new carpets or paint

These can all cause a range of lightweight symptoms like:
- Headaches
- Rashes
- Tiredness
- Poor concentration
- Blocked or runny nose
- Dry, sore eyes

But long term it can lead to more serious issues. If you find your symptoms all improve whilst on holiday, this may be an indication that your office is making you sick, although the issue could also be stress-based.

Cured meats
Cured meats like bacon and ham in days gone by were cured using salt, this is a non-toxic method of preserving meat but it is a longer process and therefore costs more money. In a bid for speed, manufacturers have started to use nitrates as a preservative and anti-bacterial. The problem with nitrates is that they have been linked to an increase in colon cancer risk.[63] It is possible to now buy nitrate-free bacon and ham.

Monosodium glutamate
It has been recognised since the '60s that this substance can harm us; the number of people who get symptoms after having eaten Chinese food has led it to be officially named 'Chinese Restaurant Syndrome'. Symptoms might be:
- Heart palpitations
- Sweating
- Flushing
- Headaches
- Numbness / tingling
- Chest pain
- Nausea

MSG is an excitotoxin which means that it can overexcite our cells to the point of damage or death. The brain cells are particularly susceptible to its effects.[64]

Plastics
One of the main problems with plastics is that they contain hormone-disrupting chemicals that are playing a part in the

increase of breast and prostate cancer levels.[65] In addition, Bisphenol A (BPA), an industrial chemical that has been used in plastics and resins since the 1960s, has been associated with increased rates of cardiovascular disease, diabetes and liver damage.[66] BPA was originally developed as a synthetic oestrogen drug, later it was polymerised (where single molecules are reacted together to form a chain of molecules) and found to be a useful substance to make plastic bottles and to coat the inside of food / drink cans and till receipts. These plastics leach oestrogen-like substances into the food and drink that they are surrounding, this is worse if the plastic is heated up (think of your plastic water bottle left in the car on a hot day, or any of the plastic containers that you might put in a microwave). The more flexible the plastic, the more it leaches these hormone disruptors, especially if the food has a fat content; it is almost impossible now to buy cheese that is not wrapped in plastic. A 2011 study showed that after testing the urine of a person who had consumed soup from a BPA-lined can, before and after, the amount of BPA in the urine increased by 1221%.[67] Canada banned the use of BPA in 2011 on the grounds of its toxicity, so it is possible to live without these substances. Cheese / meat used to be wrapped in unbleached greaseproof paper and bottles used to be made out of glass. In order to make change we need to be voting with our feet, buying glass bottles (and recycling them) and asking our food providers to use alternative packaging. I have been known to take a roll of greaseproof paper with me when I go shopping so I don't have to have my food wrapped in plastic.

Perfumes

Fragrance, an ingredient in most perfumes, is a generic term that can cover a multitude of toxins. The cosmetic industry has swung this one because they claim that their ingredients need to remain an industry secret. Ingredients range from phthalates and parabens to synthetic musks, which can disrupt hormone levels and cause cancer. The latest most ludicrous invention is scents for babies with all of these toxins in – do babies not smell delicious enough?

Sunscreen
Since the 1970s, rates of melanoma (skin cancer) have tripled, which seems a little odd when we are all becoming more diligent about sunscreen. However, when you start looking at the ingredients of most sunscreens, it might explain why. Two main toxic ingredients are Retinyl palmitate – this form of vitamin A has been linked with skin tumours and lesions – and Oxybenzone, which is a recognised hormone-disrupting chemical that can act like the hormone oestrogen. Oxybenzone is one of the chemicals that has been detected in breast milk. The other problem with slapping factor 50 on all the time is that it prevents the body from making vitamin D, the very vitamin that helps to protect us against cancer. I am not one for advocating sunburn but I think we need to get a balance here – most people can have 20–30 minutes out in the sun with no sunscreen, without burning. After that, get out of the sun or cover up. If you have a child who wants to be in the pool all day then there are sun suits or non-toxic sunscreens available – see RESOURCES. The less toxic sunscreens can be a bit more thick and gloopy, not that glide-on spray, but at least they are not toxic.

Sanitaryware
Again, manufacturers of these products have wiggled around having to disclose ingredients because these products are considered to be 'medical'. Firstly, we have the plastics in sanitary towels with all their hormone-disrupting capabilities, then we have the bleaches that are used to create our bright white tampons; these convert to dioxin-like substances, which are carcinogens and they also have hormone-

disrupting properties. Finally, if this is not enough, we then need to consider the pesticides used on the cotton that is used to create conventional tampons – see RESOURCES.

Paracetamol and other non-steroidal anti-inflammatory drugs (NSAIDS)
I know many people who pop these like sweets, often for slight symptoms, totally unaware these pain-relieving drugs can cause considerable damage to the gut wall by increasing the acidity and damaging cells,[68] this was research done back in 1987! When your body gives you pain, try to listen and discover the underlying cause rather than squashing the message and forcing the body to act as if there is nothing wrong.

Mammograms
This is the most common way that conventional medicine hopes to detect breast cancer. My concern is that we are exposing potentially cancerous tissue to radiation – exactly the substance that can cause a healthy cell to mutate into a cancerous one. In addition, the pressure that the breast tissue is being exposed to during a mammogram – the breast is squashed between two metal plates – can also damage breast tissue. If you have a tumour in your breast, the pressure can be enough to rupture the tumour, allowing the cancer cells to spread out. The other problem with mammograms is that they lead to over-diagnosis: our breasts produce lumps and bumps over our lifetime and many of them will disappear by themselves. I am not suggesting that you ignore lumps and bumps – get them checked – but they do not automatically mean that you have breast cancer. In 2000 *The Lancet* (one of the best known and oldest medical journals), having reviewed mammography, said: 'Screening for breast cancer with mammography is unjustified.'[69]

I want to be very clear here, I am NOT suggesting that we don't get screened but there are alternatives: I recommend ultrasound and thermography. The benefits of the first are that it is much more thorough (a more time-consuming and expensive service to provide, but we are talking about detecting a potential life-threatening disease). The scanner can scan right up into the armpit, somewhere that is ignored with mammograms. The benefit of thermography is that it can detect a potential tumour much earlier. For a tumour to grow to anything larger than a pinhead, it has to attract a blood supply which creates more heat and this is what a thermogram can detect. I feel very strongly that the more women put their foot down and demand to have these alternative screening methods, the more the NHS will have to start listening but we need the numbers to make a difference.

My thermogram story
At the age of 49 I received my letter inviting me to have a mammogram and I had agreed with myself that, when that letter arrived, I would start having thermograms, so I got in touch with Medical Thermal Imaging (MTI) and booked in. I skipped along to the appointment assuming that there would be nothing wrong. I was aware that I had a tendency to be oestrogen dominant – my genetics showed that the liver pathway responsible for detoxing oestrogen had mutations on it) – so I was doing lots of liver support and taking a supplement called DIM which helps your liver to process extra oestrogen. This, however, did not turn out to be quite enough and the results were not as hunky dory as I would have liked. When your results are assessed you are given a grading, this is TH1 to TH5:

TH1 and 2 are considered good, everything is normal.

TH3 is considered questionable but not abnormal, very often the situation can have normalised by the time you have your next scan but it is important to keep scanning.

TH4 and TH5 are considered abnormal with a higher risk. Action needs to be taken here to balance things up.

On my right breast I was TH3 and on my left breast I was TH4 – I have to say I was a little freaked out until I talked to the wonderful Rosa at MTI who was incredibly reassuring and armed me with a whole host of further things that I could be doing to balance up my hormones and improve the situation. There were other supplements that I could take and neuro-lymphatic breast massage that I could do – have a look on YouTube for Prune Harris – *Balancing the Breasts*, it is a 3-minute video to show you how to do this. It is important to remember to actually do these things on a daily basis, something I often struggle with when introducing a new habit. I have to link it to an activity that I do every day so for this one I do it whilst waiting for our dogs to finish their breakfast (one of our dogs has problems with sticking to her own bowl so some supervision is necessary). The fact that my left breast was worse, correlated perfectly with the fact that my root canal was on the left side of my mouth, if you have a root canal I urge you to watch the film *Root Cause*. Apologies, I know that I am repeating myself but the correlation between root canal treatment and breast cancer is extremely high.[70]

Another thing that I discussed with Rosa is the emotional impact on our physiology, and she pointed me in the direction of the work of Dr Hamer. Dr Hamer discovered that after scanning the brain and organs of cancer patients and taking a history, all cancers are related to a 'serious, acute-dramatic and isolating conflict-shock experience which can be seen as lesions in the brain with a CT scan'. This lesion in the brain can correlate with an organ, and in my case my conflict was manifesting in the left breast. Dr Hamer explains that if a mother has conflict with a child it will stimulate milk production by increasing the number of breast cells and it will cause lesions in a specific part of her right brain. My 'conflict' is that my daughter has had ME for 4½ years, this is her story so not something I can expand upon in this book, but I will say that it has been one of the most challenging times in my life and a huge learning curve. If the mother is right-handed, the lesion in the brain will be on the right side, this in turn relates to the left breast. I had some work to do regarding separating myself from my daughter's struggles. In my line of work it is hard not to try to 'fix' everybody, I had been trying to do this for my daughter and the realisation that I had to stop taking responsibility for her illness and hand that over to her (she is after all now 20 and an adult) was more than liberating. This is an ongoing process, however – ceasing to take responsibility for your child's ill health is challenging to say the least, but I am getting there.

If you want to look more into the subject of mammograms and breast cancer screening, there is a very well-referenced documentary called *The Promise*.

Whilst we are on women's health, I would just like to bring up the topic of the HPV vaccine. Vaccination is a very contentious subject and it is not my intention to get embroiled in the subject in this book but what I will just mention is that in Japan they have stopped promoting the use of the HPV vaccine due to the high number of Adverse Drug Reactions that were occurring in young girls, ranging from nausea and vomiting to seizures and paralysis.[71]

Dry cleaners

Perchloroethylene, more commonly known as PERC, is the most commonly used solvent in dry cleaning fluids. Studies show that there is a link between this substance and the increased risk of cancers.[72] If you work in a dry cleaners, take protective measures and talk to the boss about ways to decrease exposure and increase ventilation. If you collect your clothes from the dry cleaners, remove the plastic and hang them outside for a couple of hours to air.

Nail varnish / gel nails
It stands to reason that something that comes in every colour of the rainbow and smells, to say the least, unnatural is going to contain toxins. Usually it is the toxic trio: formaldehyde, toluene and dibutyl phthalate. Yes, formaldehyde that is used to preserve dead bodies and is a known carcinogen, toluene which is the chemical in many glues, and can cause cardiac arrest.[73] Dibutyl pthalate can cause developmental defects and affect fertility, it is also a plasticiser used in children's toys! Think of all those young people working in nail bars inhaling that stuff all day, and just because you are putting it on your nails don't think that the chemicals cannot be absorbed through the nail bed. It is possible to buy non-toxic nail varnish – see RESOURCES.

Spray tan
This contains DHA – dihydroxyacetone, a mild to moderate toxin, but one which, when sprayed and inhaled, can cause damage to DNA, leading to cancer. If you need to have a spray tan try to get it rubbed on rather than sprayed, and there are also far less toxic self-tanners – see RESOURCES.

Hair dye
The most toxic compound in hair dye is para-phenylene-diamine, and studies show an increased risk for cancer in people who use permanent hair dye.[74] Confession – this is one toxin that I have not managed to remove from my life, and I knowingly apply it every 4–6 weeks. My self-esteem does not stretch far enough to revert to my natural colour, a mousey brown with grey bits in it, although I have sourced the least toxic one that I can find – see RESOURCES.

Tuna and other mercury-containing fish
Tuna, swordfish, king mackerel, marlin and shark. I have some clients who are having a tuna sandwich every day,

believing this is a healthy option because they are eating lots of oily fish. The larger the fish, the more likely it is to accumulate heavy metals and toxins. In 1956 in Japan a factory was pumping out high levels of mercury waste, and the local population started to get really sick, muscle weakness, an inability to walk, convulsions, paralysis and sometimes coma. The levels are obviously not that high in the fish that we eat today, but it all adds to the toxic load. Better types of oily fish are mackerel (these are small not like the king mackerel), salmon, sardines, anchovies and herring – it goes without saying not the farmed variety which are grown in such cramped conditions they require pesticides and antibiotics to keep disease levels under control. If you compare a portion of farmed and wild salmon you can see the huge difference: besides the overall colour, the farmed salmon has white stripes of fat in it – the fat is where most of the toxins in a body will be stored. If you are interested have a look at the *Fillet Oh Fish* documentary on YouTube which gives some alarming insights into farmed fish.

Non-stick pans
Teflon, that non-stick coating that makes washing up so easy, is toxic enough to kill a canary in the kitchen. When Teflon is heated it releases 6 different toxic chemicals, some of which cause cancer but others cause the lungs of birds to haemorrhage.[75] For humans it can do harm in the same way but just to a lesser extent. The really disturbing thing is that Teflon is being used as a substance in school uniforms to make them stain resistant.

Aluminium foil
Aluminium is toxic to the brain and nervous system,[76] in particular it has been associated with Alzheimer's.

***

Apologies, I did forewarn you that it is a rather depressing picture. All of these things per se are not going to have you instantly sick after one exposure, unless your body has got to an extremely damaged state where it has no resilience, but the cumulative exposure over years means that the toxic load is overwhelming.

WE JUST DON'T KNOW

Many chemicals are tested and deemed 'safe'; however, there are two problems with this approach, firstly they are being tested on an adult-sized body – what about our children? The Environmental Working Group (EWG) took blood samples from the cord blood of newborn babies and recorded 232 toxic chemicals in them, ranging from fire retardants, chemical fragrances to detergents and PFBA – non-stick coating. No wonder there are so many children presenting with autism and ADHD: their brains are being poisoned so that they cannot develop properly. The second problem with the testing of chemicals is the interaction between them. Chemicals are tested separately and may pass the test, but if you start mixing these chemicals up and analysing their interactions I am sure that you would start to see very different types of results that would make your toes curl.

SIGNS AND SYMPTOMS THAT MAY MEAN YOU ARE OVER-TOXIC AND YOUR LIVER NEEDS SOME TLC

- Headaches
- Feeling hungover when you haven't been drinking
- Pain just under the ribs or between the shoulder blades
- Itchy skin
- Indigestion
- Low tolerance to alcohol – e.g. getting drunk quickly

- Diarrhoea
- Bloating
- Constipation
- Gallstones
- Bad breath – not just a bit of morning bad breath – proper halitosis
- Nausea
- Loss of energy, although there can be a multitude of reasons for this
- Indigestion after fatty food
- Stiff achey muscles

You may have done a liver function test and it has come back clear but a liver function test only really shows up when there is proper dysfunction. For me it is important to listen to the rumblings of the body before they start turning into something more serious. If you are showing some of the above signs / symptoms then it would be a good idea to give your liver some attention.

There is no easy answer to the toxins issue, as it is impossible to seal ourselves off from the environment. I hope that as time goes on and we all become more aware of these dangers that things will start to change. In the meantime, however, as it is not possible to all live in the Outer Hebrides surviving off the land, below are some of my suggestions.

Where possible eat organic – EWG is a very useful website if you want to check ingredients of foods etc, they also do a useful Dirty Dozen printout for foods that are exposed to higher levels of pesticides and herbicides and a Clean Fifteen for the less toxic fruits and vegetables.

Use toxin-free toiletries – that includes soap, shampoo, conditioner, deodorant, shaving cream, toothpaste, make-up etc. See RESOURCES for good ethical companies. Be aware that there are companies claiming that their products are organic / toxin-free when they are not.

Try not to cook with non-stick pans, use stainless steel cookware or ceramic – Green Pan sell a good range.

Try not to put aluminium foil directly onto food – use greaseproof paper over it or, if you want to make a foil parcel, line it with greaseproof paper. Most ready-made meals will come in aluminium trays and aluminium is also contained in most anti-perspirants and deodorants.

Clingfilm – if you need to cover food buy silicon food covers or the beeswax organic reusable food wraps. If you have to use clingfilm and it is going to touch the food put a layer of greaseproof between the food and the clingfilm so there is no direct contact.

Try not to use plastic water bottles – buy stainless steel ones. See RESOURCES. If you can, buy bottled water in glass bottles – also much better for the environment if you recycle.

Try to source flame-retardant-free goods, e.g. soft furnishings and fabrics. It is possible to find chemical-free fire-retardant treated fabrics – see RESOURCES.

EMR – HOW TO REDUCE YOUR EXPOSURE

Wherever you can in the home, get your computers hard-wired so you don't need wifi. If this is not possible, make sure that you turn your wifi off at night, if you are the sort of person like me who will forget, put it on a timer. And even in the day if you don't need it. I am aware that if you live in a built-up area, even if you turn your own wifi off you will probably be getting everyone else's. Perhaps you could set up a local neighbourhood scheme for everyone to turn off their wifi at night; I have been made aware of the issue that if people turn off their wifi at night the providers lower the bandwidth, so make sure that the providers are aware of what your neighbourhood is doing.

Try to keep your phone in airplane mode as much as

possible. For the times where this is not practical keep your phone as far away from your body as you can – at least half a metre. If you are talking on the phone, use loud speaker or headphones, ideally an airtube headset (stops any potential EMR running up the metal wire) with an integrated microphone so you don't have to hold your phone. It is particularly difficult for our younger generation with FOMO (fear of missing out) issues: they seem to need to be permanently attached, there are now bras being sold with phone pockets in!!! Disaster. We need to educate our young and get them into using airplane mode – perhaps someone will develop a phone that automatically switches into airplane mode when not in use.

Keep your use of Bluetooth devices to an absolute minimum – this includes fitness trackers. Make sure that if you are using one it is one where you can turn off the Bluetooth and only turn it on for syncing data.

Try not to use your laptop on your lap – put it on a table. I used to find if I sat with my iPad on my knee my legs would go fuzzy.

Try not to take your phone / iPad into the bedroom.

Try not to use your phone when the reception is bad, for every bar that is missing your exposure increases.

When using your phone in the car i.e. a big metal box which magnifies the radiation, keep it on airplane mode unless you need to make a call. Listen to podcasts / music etc that you have already downloaded.

DETOXING

Detoxing unfortunately has gained the reputation of being rather faddish, but if you look at detoxing over time, various methods have been practised for centuries.

Sweating – either with exercise or sauna, this is a great way for the liver to detox as it can get rid of excess toxins through the skin. It is important that you shower as soon as possible after you have been sweating – do this with cold water to shut the pores and prevent reabsorption – you can then have a nice hot shower after. Also make sure that you are drinking lots of clean water.

Infra-red saunas – these are saunas that use light to create heat, this means that it can penetrate the body more effectively. Infra-red light is emitted from the sun all of the time but it is not damaging like the ultra-violet rays. Having just talked about the damage that EMR can do to the body, infra-red saunas produce EMR on the spectrum that is beneficial to the body – perhaps some clever scientist out there could work out a way of running our electrical devices on this spectrum of EMR. This spectrum of beneficial EMR helps to trigger the parasympathetic nervous system (this is your rest and digest one), and studies have shown that infra-red treatment can improve depression and anxiety.[77] It also increases your heart rate and blood flow,[78] which can decrease inflammation. I have an infra-red sauna pod at home which I sit in with my head sticking out – sometimes with a woolly hat on in the winter if my bedroom is cold. It helps me heat up quicker and also is more evidence for my family that I have completely lost the plot and probably need to be committed.

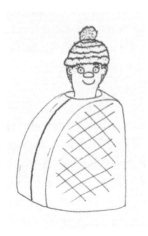

Exercising – the lymph system is made up of lots of lymph vessels like the blood vessel system; however, it does not have the luxury of a heart to pump the lymph around, it relies on muscle contraction. The lymph system, as well as being a vital part of our immune system, also helps to carry toxins out of the body.

Body brushing – this stimulates the circulation to flow, helping the detox process. There is also anecdotal evidence that it helps to clear cellulite, which would make sense as cellulite tends to form on areas of the body where there is the least circulation. Use firm upward strokes – it is OK to make the skin a bit pink but don't be too brutal!

Enemas – now this is where everyone tends to get a bit squeamish and, yes, I do partake of these myself when I am feeling keen or a bit yucky – you know that slightly hungover feeling in the morning that you can get even when you haven't been drinking. They are much easier to perform than you would think. Enemas are not a new invention, they have been around for centuries; in Henry VIII's time, he employed a Groom of the Stool who performed regular enemas to keep the royal bowel squeaky clean. Though a practice with a long history, sadly they have been lost from mainstream practices as we become more and more sanitary. Coffee enemas in particular can stimulate bile flow in the liver, which helps to speed up the detoxification process. Enema kits are very easy to get hold of. See RESOURCES. If you can't face doing it yourself book in for some colonic irrigation.

Gut health – ensure that you have good gut health, pathogenic bacteria produce toxins and if your gut is leaky these will be leaking straight into the bloodstream.

Liver support – supporting your liver function is vital for a successful detox. The liver is the most important detox organ and it gets a serious work-out in our modern-day world. It removes all substances that are foreign to the human body or excessive levels of endogenous substances i.e. things that naturally occur in the body, like hormones. This is quite a feat and there are many ways that we can help the liver to do its job.

Foods that support liver function are:
Cruciferous vegetables – broccoli, kale, Brussels sprouts, cauliflower, cabbage, bok choi and kohlrabi.

Sulphurous foods – eggs, onions, garlic, leeks, asparagus and chives.

Natural supplements that can support liver function are milk thistle, dandelion and turmeric.

Keeping blood sugar levels balanced also helps the liver so that it does not have to spend too much time converting sugar into fat.

Look after your kidneys, these are also an important detox organ.

Make sure that you are drinking enough water – see below.

Foods to support kidney function are parsley, dandelion, ginger, nettle, turmeric and celery.

Reduce caffeine and alcohol.

Water or juice fasting – never a popular suggestion but it does wonders for your body and I assure you that it is really not as bad as it sounds. Every year I take a group of people juicing for a week in Malta: the newbies are often quite understandably nervous at the prospect of no food for a week but the comments when we get out there are 'This really isn't too bad' and 'I don't feel hungry at all.' When we fast, we give our digestive system a break, which means that we lighten the load on the liver and it can increase rates of detoxing, clearing out those stored toxins from fat cells, joints and wherever else it has packed them away because it couldn't deal with them at the time. These juice retreats also involve colonic hydrotherapy (not compulsory but highly recommended) and lymphatic drainage massage, as well as lots of sunshine, relaxation, yoga and conversations about bowel movements.

Water – make sure that you are well hydrated. To work out the daily amount of water that you should be drinking in litres for your body, multiply your weight in kgs by 0.033. If you are doing a lot of sweating add a bit more. Try to drink filtered water. Tea and coffee do not count towards your hydration but herbal tea does. Many people turn their noses up at the idea of herbal tea but search around: there is such a huge variety I feel sure there is something out there for everyone. Red bush tea is the closest thing I have found to black tea, although it can be a bit of a love it or hate it thing. If you are drinking well below the recommended amount then increase your water consumption slowly – give the body time to get used to it. You are likely to pee quite a lot to start with but then everything will settle down.

ALCOHOL

Whilst we are on the subject of drinks, it would be remiss of me not to include alcohol, a socially acceptable toxin; however, I am not an advocate of teetotalism. In the words of a famous physician, Li Shizhen of the Ming dynasty, who lived in the 16th century:

'Wine is indeed a delicious drink bestowed by Heaven. Drinking it properly helps the blood and qi circulate, invigorates the mind, eases mental stress, and adds to the pleasure of life. Drinking without restraint impairs the mind, the blood and the stomach qi, producing internal heat which leads at best to disease and at worst to the humiliation of the nation, the ruin of the family and the loss of life!'

There is evidence to show that moderate drinkers live longer than teetotalers, I am not sure of the reason for this, it may be the antioxidants in wine but my personal view is that there is huge value in sitting down at the end of the day with a glass of something and having that aaaarrrhhhh moment, switching off from the day. However, I am talking about ONE glass of something and not every night. Also, this has to be tailored to the individual. When we look at our individual liver detox ability, alcohol is processed more efficiently by some people than others, so you will have to listen to your body on this one. Another issue surrounding alcohol is sulfites, which are the preservatives in many wines. Some people who can't tolerate wine are reacting to the sulfites – I include myself in that category. In a bid to not feel rough the next day I have found that vodka is my best tipple: a delicious skinny bitch cocktail (vodka, lots of fresh lime juice and sparkling water) slips down a treat with no long-term adverse effects. Vodka is one of the cleanest forms of alcohol (and generally has better results than gin, which can have you crying in the corner), lower in sugar than many other alcohols as long as you are careful about your mixer – no coke / lemonade!

A WORD ABOUT WEIGHT-LOSS
If you are trying to lose weight and your body is really toxic, a favourite place for the liver to store toxins is in the fat cells (cellulite). In order for the body to break down fat cells it has to be able to cope with the toxins that are going to be released. An important part of successful weight-loss is really supporting liver function and being aware of reducing your toxic exposure.

I apologise for writing such a depressing chapter but I feel it is important to forearm you. Don't despair, as you can see there are a huge array of things that we can do to help protect ourselves. In addition, as the groundswell of public opinion grows, we will hopefully be able to eradicate many of these toxins from our environment so that there is less for us to protect ourselves against.

8

STRESS

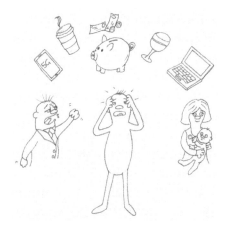

'You can't stop the waves but you can learn to surf.'
— Jon Kabat-Zinn

This is the big one, the thing that I spend most of my time helping clients with. I would estimate that 95% of my clients have a disordered stress response and it is usually the factor that most affects their health. The perception that the body and mind are separate entities is a completely misguided paradigm. Every single cell in the body has receptors on their cell membranes that respond to neurotransmitters (brain chemicals). So every thought and feeling that we have impacts every single cell in the body. In consultations, stress comes in all shapes and sizes: a totally wired client who could not sit for longer than 10 minutes during a 90-minute consultation, leaping up to pace around the room, to a client whose whole body visibly started shaking when he began telling me about relations with various members of his family … and then come the copious tears that fall as the clients start to offload their heavy burdens. 'Better out than in' is always my motto; the amount of apologies from clients I receive as they release their emotions is a sign of our society's repressive rules and stiff-upper-lip attitude, which makes us feel that it is not OK to express ourselves fully.

Allowing our bodies to run chronic stress is probably the single most damaging thing that we can do to it, and boy have I managed to fall into this category. The good news is that there is a huge amount that can be done to teach the body to turn off its stress response, so don't despair.

Our physical stress response is quite simply out of date: we are still running on the principle that governed us for thousands of years whilst we were living in caves. Stress then, meant a life-threatening situation – bumping into a sabre-toothed tiger or woolly mammoth. In our current world, don't get me wrong, this still serves us on the very rare occasions that we might nearly get run over by a bus or on a more regular basis for our valiant soldiers in a combat situation, but generally day to day this physical response is completely out of proportion. In a world with faster communication, we are being constantly bombarded with information, to which we feel the need to react. This lack of stillness makes it feel as if time is going faster and faster, and there are simply not enough minutes in the day to accomplish all the things that we want or feel that we need to do. This sense of overwhelm can be relentless, resulting in the body constantly feeling under threat. Although many of our modern current stresses can feel as if they are life-threatening, they are not, making our exaggerated physical response unnecessary.

WHAT HAPPENS WHEN THE FIGHT / FLIGHT RESPONSE
IS TRIGGERED?

1. the adrenals kick into action
The adrenals produce adrenalin, which gets everything pumped up and on alert for that life-threatening danger. They also produce cortisol; this has the effect of putting more sugar into the bloodstream to travel to the muscles, providing energy for our fighting or running. The trouble with this is that rarely do we burn that sugar off. With modern-day stress, we are more likely to be sitting in a traffic jam, late for a meeting, or sitting at our desk sweating over a deadline or phone call. That damaging sugar needs to be dealt with quickly by the production of insulin. Insulin goes around in the bloodstream asking the cells to take up the excess sugar, however, if our cells have started to become insulin resistant (see SUGAR Chapter) the body has to send the sugar to the liver where it is converted into fat. This fat is deposited around the middle and in amongst the abdominal organs, making us more apple-shaped.

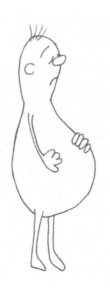

The difference between fat around the middle (visceral fat) and other fat (subcutaneous fat):

Subcutaneous fat is mostly inactive and serves as an insulator and a source of energy if needed.

Visceral fat is much more active amd makes a whole host of chemical messengers that in high levels are unhelpful. These are:

Blood clotting agents – increasing the risk for heart attacks and strokes.

Hormones that constrict our blood vessels and lead to raised blood pressure.

Agents that increase inflammation by triggering the body's immune system unnecessarily.

Excess oestrogen in men as well as women which promotes cancer.

Helpful and unhelpful measurements:
Measuring someone's BMI (body mass index) is not necessarily that useful. This is a measurement of someone's height to weight ratio, so you divide your weight in kgs by your height in metres. These are the guidelines for BMI:
- 18.5 or below – underweight
- 18.5–24.9 – healthy weight
- 25–29.9 – overweight
- 30 and above – obese

The problem with this calculation is that if you imagine a rugby player who is solid muscle, which weighs much more than fat, his BMI will say that he is in the obese bracket. A much more helpful measurement is hip to waist ratio to see if you are carrying excess weight around the middle. For this you measure the circumference of your hips at the widest part of your buttocks and then your waist – your natural waist usually is just above the belly button. You then divide the waist measurement by your hip measurement. For optimal health women's should be less than 0.8 and for men it should be less than 0.95.

Back to the adrenals, if we are constantly requiring the adrenal glands to produce cortisol, the adrenals can start to show signs of fatigue; the types of symptoms that you might experience if this is happening are:

Unrelenting tiredness or fatigue

Feeling tired but wired

Cravings for sugar

Cravings for salt

Dizziness upon standing

Heart palpitations

Feeling weak, shaky, dizzy, irritable if you don't eat regularly

Feeling drowsy after a meal, especially if it contains carbs/sugar

Low blood pressure

Mental fogginess

Low tolerance to exercise

Difficulty getting out of bed in the morning

Need to start the day with caffeine

More energy in the evening

Sleep issues – either struggling to drop off to sleep or waking in the middle of the night with a whizzy mind

Regular illness at weekends or when you go on holiday

Inability to handle stress generally

Panic attacks or being easily startled

Memory loss

Low immune function – you tend to catch everything going

Hormone imbalance

Depression

Imbalanced adrenal function is a hugely common problem, which I see with the majority of my clients; unfortunately it is not something that is generally recognised by the medical profession unless you have Addison's or Cushing's disease (these are diseases where the cortisol levels are so low or high that it can be life-threatening). Many of the above symptoms are down to blood sugar levels swinging up and down. See FOOD Chapter for foods to help balance blood sugar levels.

2. increased blood pressure

Our pulse rate and blood pressure go up to get more blood round the body to oxygenate the muscles for our fighting and flighting. Our blood vessels constrict, which means that the extra pressure can cause damage to the blood vessel wall or even cause an aneurism (where the blood vessel ruptures). If it is a little blood vessel you won't notice but it is still causing damage and inflammation in the body; obviously if it is a bigger blood vessel this can have serious long-term or even short-term life-threatening effects.

3. suppressed immune system

It is not important that you fight the bacterial infection in your big toe when you are in life-threatening combat. The implications of this are huge as we are all being exposed to bacterial / viral infections on a constant basis. Many of us suffer from low grade infections which don't exactly floor us but have a slow insidious effect on our energy levels and general wellbeing. Viruses like Epstein-Barr can manifest in full-blown glandular fever, but they can also exist in the system without giving overt symptoms, just running us down. There are a huge number of different viruses that our bodies are exposed to regularly and the immune system needs to be strong to fight them off. If you are not feeling right and you have been to the doctor and all the tests come back negative (most viral infections don't show up on conventional blood tests) it may well be that you have a virus that is draining the system. Reducing the stress response as well as nourishing the body and reducing sugar can go a long way to boosting the immune system and helping it get these viruses under control. Having a fully functioning ninja immune system is vital, particularly with regard to detecting and eradicating cancer cells.

4. suppressed regeneration and repair
Our body is constantly regenerating and repairing tissue; if you are in mortal combat this is not a priority, so many of the housekeeping jobs get put on the back burner and long term you can develop conditions like leaky gut and osteoporosis where the bones are not being properly maintained.

5. suppressed digestion
Digestion takes up a huge amount of energy but again it is not a priority that your eggs and bacon are broken down and absorbed properly when your life is in danger. Long-term suppression of digestive function leads to nutrient deficiencies, which can have a profound effect on the entire body.

6. increased acidity
Excess cortisol in the system means that your body will be more acidic and so you lose extra magnesium and potassium in the urine. Both of these alkalising minerals help to maintain the pH in the body. Symptoms of excess acidity can be chronic muscle pain, headaches, Chronic Fatigue, irritability and panic attacks.

7. musculoskeletal issues
When the body and the muscles are tense, this can lead to muscle pains and the skeleton being pulled out of line. This

can then lead to more muscle pain but it can also restrict the nerves and the function of the organ that this nerve is connected to.

8. overworked liver
High levels of blood sugar that are not being used up means that the liver is constantly spending time and energy on converting sugar from the bloodstream into fat, when it has many other duties to perform, most importantly detoxing and assimilation of nutrients.

9. changes the shape of your brain
The part of your brain that detects stress and stores fear memories is the amygdala; if it is being constantly stimulated it starts to increase in size. The hippocampus, positioned right beside the amygdala, helps us to regulate memory and emotions and if there are high levels of cortisol in the system the communication between the amygdala and the hippocampus becomes hard-wired. This means that we are much more predisposed to be in a state of fight / flight, overreacting to things that we normally wouldn't. The hippocampus is also responsible for maturing stem cells into brain cells and if there is a state of chronic stress this function is reduced – it might explain why chronic stress adversely affects memory and learning. And if that is not enough, excess cortisol also shrinks the prefrontal cortex, the area of the brain that is responsible for concentration, judgement, decision-making and social interaction. Due to the wonderful neuroplasticity (think plasticine, the brain is very malleable and adaptable) of the brain, this process is reversible but it is imperative that the cortisol levels are reduced for the repair process to start.

If all of the above is not enough, when the body is exposed to stress, be it a chemical, physical or biological threat, each individual cell employs a cell danger response (CDR). This is a metabolic response to try and maintain balance by

protecting and conserving a cell's resources. The CDR
affects / causes:

The flow of electrons, which means that there is increased oxidation – a prime cause of ageing.

Reduced oxygen consumption – a lack of oxygen causes
cell death.

Reduced fluidity of the cell membrane – substances cannot move in and out of the cell so efficiently.

Reduced ability of cell to 'traffic' metals; it is vital that
cells maintain an optimal level of metals to regulate the
internal environment of the cell.

Altered lipid dynamics – lipid (fat) droplets within the
cell are vital for communication between different organelles within the cell.

Reduced vitamin availability.

Reduced ability of the proteins in DNA to fold correctly
– leading to DNA mutation.

When the CDR is employed for abnormal amounts of
time, it is easy to understand why organ function starts to
go 'wrong', which then results in chronic disease.

GENETICS CAN MAKE YOU MORE STRESS PRONE

People with mutations on the COMT gene can be slow to
process the stress hormones out of the system; this means
that they hang around and extend the stress response. I have
these mutations but I am not allowing this to become an
excuse for my stress, it just means that I have to be a little
bit more diligent about my homework and how I choose to
respond to events in life.

STRESS CAN BECOME A BODY HABIT

When your adrenals get used to constantly running in the
'wired' zone, this can then become preprogammed, to make

it more straightforward. At the end of the day our body is trying to be as efficient as possible. If we run stress a lot it can become the default mode of operation, the pathways that run the stress reaction become very efficient so that it is actually easier for the body to run stress than relaxation. If our bodies had been designed for 21st-century living, we might have been blessed with an off-switch for the stress response.

Taking all of this into consideration, if we live in a state of chronic stress, it is not surprising that body biochemistry goes haywire and develops chronic disease. This is one of the most complex issues that I address with clients; for many the diet change is easy enough, the exercise can be done no problem ... but address the lifestyle, change attitudes to life events and create enough stillness and security for the fight / flight mechanism to switch itself off? Now that can be a great challenge.

For some clients it is enough to balance adrenal function by making sure they are keeping their blood sugar levels even, are aware of their stress and perhaps practise some mindfulness and meditation. However, for those clients who may have had a more profound experience and have been carrying it since childhood this simply is not enough. I hesitate to use the word trauma, because for most people the word trauma conjures up the more extreme events – sexual abuse, combat experiences, bereavement, constant parental rejection... But trauma can come in all shapes and sizes, especially when we are children and we do not have the capacity to process experiences with the wisdom and emotional intelligence that we may have gained in adulthood. Trauma could be:

Your mother having a really bad day and being disproportionately impatient with you.

A frustrated older sibling saying 'When we get home, I'm going to kill you.'

Your father giving you a smack (perhaps the one and only smack that he ever gave you).

Your teacher standing you up in front of the whole school and humiliating you.

Your pet dying.

Being forced to finish what is on your plate.

I am not necessarily saying that one of these events will traumatise with lifelong effects ... but it could. Often a combination of ongoing experiences that challenge the feeling of security for a child can set up a lifetime of insecurity, where the body is constantly on the alert for danger.

In these situtions a bit of adrenal support and breathing is not going to cut the mustard – we are looking at reprogramming a lifetime's learnt behaviour of scanning for danger in order to keep us safe. For these people it is nearly impossible to sit and relax without feeling that you should be doing something, and there is often a panic at the sight of a gap in the diary. I know that I can start to feel very twitchy if there is a space in my day. My brain starts to scan for jobs to fill the gap and of course there are always jobs to fill that gap, whether it is important that they are done now is immaterial to a stress-head.

Let me talk you through my day when I was running the stress programme:

Wake up, and in my experience my heart would start pounding immediately as my thoughts kicked in with the enormity of my to-do list. This got me bouncing out of bed because I had adrenalin and cortisol in the system. Stress-heads are usually constantly scanning their environment and permanently have thoughts whirring around in their heads. If you manage to sit down to eat breakfast you will be busy reading the back of the cereal packet / newspaper, listening to the news, jumping up to do just that thing that can't possibly wait because you might forget to do it later – what is wrong with just eating! A stress-head will look at their watch 5 minutes before they need to leave on the school run or for work and think 'Oh five minutes, can't waste that I'll just do X', X usually takes longer than 5 minutes and so you then end up being late for work / school run, yelling at the children, having heart palpitations because you get stuck behind a learner driver and the traffic lights are always on red. The day will be packed back to back, every minute accounted for with 'achievement'. Lunch if there is time will be crammed in whilst doing emails, putting a wash on or walking the dog. You end up doing things for your children that they are quite capable of doing themselves because it is easier and quicker and of course you wish to be a popular loveable mummy. A wise friend said to me that every time you do something for your children that they are quite capable of doing themsleves you are mentally disabling them! That brought me up short, now when I am being a helicopter mother to my grown-up children, they will quote this back at me. You get through to the end of the day, have your evening meal and when you should be having some downtime, that little voice kicks in again 'well you could just get that done' – so tempting, it means one less job tomorrow or if you do manage to sit down and perhaps watch some TV you just go fast asleep and miss it all.

I think you get the picture. We create lives for ourselves where there just isn't a minute for anything to not 'go to plan' and if there is a hitch, it throws out the timetable which is inordinately stressful because we are no longer in control and having to play catch-up. It also does not leave much room for FUN, but more on that later.

In practise I see lots of different variations of this type of overwhelming existence, my job is to try and create some space for the client. When I talk to clients about creating space they often say 'But where, there just isn't room for me.' The thing is, it doesn't take much extra time for you, what is really key is *how* you approach the busyness of your life. You can have two people who are in exactly the same situations, but one is wired on the ceiling about it and the other is a zen god / goddess.

BEHAVIOURAL SIGNS THAT YOU MIGHT BE STRESSED
Lost your sense of humour – humour is a hugely valuable stress buster and an immune booster, so losing it is detrimental to your health as well as making you a not very fun person to be around.

You fly off the handle at the smallest thing – that stress pathway is quick to kick in when you run it regularly.

More impatient – *I just haven't got time for this.*

Take things too personally – often assume there is criticism when there really isn't.

Biting your nails.

Picking at your skin.

Increased alcohol consumption.

Increased sugar consumption.

Loss of libido – if you are in a life-threatening situation how can it possibly be safe to think about sex or bringing a baby into the world.

Teeth grinding – official name bruxism. Waking up with an aching / tight jaw or dull headache can be a sign of grinding your teeth at night – ask your dentist to check this, he will be able to tell if you are. You can get mouth guards to protect your teeth at night but this approach is not really solving the underlying problem of why you are grinding in the first place. I used to grind my teeth and once I became aware of it found that being aware of what I was doing with my jaw in the day was really helpful. I would often find myself driving along with my jaw tightly clenched. Making a conscious effort to relax it and massaging all around the jaw area at night can help, but reducing your stress load is the most effective strategy.

Not wanting to socialise as much – stress can make us very introverted.

How to become the Zen Master

The most important thing to realise is that switching off your fight / flight does not happen overnight, it takes a lot of homework and it takes vigilance and perseverance. If your body has got used to constantly scanning for the sabre-toothed tiger it is not suddenly going to switch itself off and chill in a deck-chair. Those stress hormones will kick in at the drop of a hat, be patient and reassuring to your body that, whatever has got it going, it is most unlikely to be threatening your very existence, although it may feel like it.

One thing I found really important to take on board:

Stress is only in the eye of the beholder

Shakespeare puts it perfectly:

'... there is nothing either good or bad, but thinking makes it so.'

We ALWAYS have a choice. I found this a rather annoying realisation – I was now going to have to take full responsibility for my reactions to anything. No longer could I blame it on my parents, siblings, husband, children, dogs, horses or the fact that I chose to take a call 5 minutes before I needed to leave for the school run. Part of my problem is that I don't like hanging out with myself, it brings a rather uncomfortable, uneasy emotion with it ... so much easier to be constantly busy. I also need to be needed, let's try and make myself indispensable so everyone will love me. So often I have put my needs on the back burner in order to not rock the boat. Sound familiar? For more on this see the SPIRIT Chapter.

If you are someone who has got to the state of permanent fight / flight with that 'overwhelm' feeling kicking in on a regular basis, and your mind is always whizzing with all of those jobs that you have to get done, and there are simply not enough hours in the day to do them, then these are a few things that might help.

Breathing
This is the most effective way to switch off the fight / flight mechanism. If we sit quietly and take our pulse, we will notice that on the in-breath our pulse rate will go slightly faster than on the out-breath. There are two sides to our nervous system, one of them, the sympathetic (fight / flight), is engaged when we are breathing in, the other side, the parasympathetic (rest and digest) is engaged when we breathe out. So, if we can extend the outbreath (approximately in for 4 and out for 8) we are helping to switch our bodies into parasympathetic, rest and digest dominance. Play around with it so it suits you, some people need to start with in for 4 and out for 6 and some can get to in for 4 and out for 16 but don't force it – it is supposed to be relaxing you! Whenever you start to feel that rising panic / anxiety / overwhelm just take 5 long, slow breaths and say to yourself 'this is not life-threatening.' Obviously if you are being chased down a dark alley by a machete-wielding madperson this may not be the ideal approach, but remembering to breathe might help your brain to work more effectively.

To help you with this type of breathing it is important to make sure that you are breathing properly. I know it sounds ridiculous, we are all breathing 24 / 7, surely we all have it cracked by now, but I find that many of my clients have lost the ability to breathe correctly. If we place one hand over our chest and one hand over our tummy and take a sharp breath in, the hand over our chest should not move, all the movement should be in the hand covering the tummy. When our tummy hand is rising it means that we are breathing deep into the diaphragm, and that we are getting much more air into the system for our long relaxing out-breath. If you struggle with this, lie on the floor with your hands placed on your tummy and practise filling the balloon. Ideally this is the way that we should be breathing all of the time and it is well worth developing the habit. If you watch a newborn baby, they breath perfectly, their little tummies rise and fall, a joy to behold before the stresses of life start to take a hold. When I started to retrain my breathing, I had an activity that I did regularly through the day as my trigger to remind me to check my breathing (mine was going to the loo) or set a pinger on your phone to ping at you every hour or so. I then did 5 slow mindful breaths to retrain.

Our breathing rate is linked to emotional states; experiments show that if you consciously breathe fast and shallow you can generate the feelings of increased anxiety, the same goes for the opposite, breathing slow and deep helps to calm the body.

Lists
Firstly, do not constantly run the to-do list in your head. Write those jobs down – write lists or dictate them to your phone – the idea is to get those jobs *out* of your head. Often we can have lots of jobs whizzing round in our heads, and that feels totally overwhelming, but as soon as we write them down there may only be 5 or 6 and it feels more manageable. A very important lesson that I have learnt and it took me a little while to catch on, is that I will NEVER get to the end of my list of jobs, however quickly I tick them off they will keep adding on the bottom.

So, what to do – I look at my list in the morning, decide how many I am going to get done (trying to be realistic) and then when done, that is ENOUGH, now it is time for me, the rest of the jobs can wait till tomorrow. This approach takes some discipline as my little voice will kick in with 'you could just fit one more job in', but I have to be strong-willed and tell it where to go – I have shut up shop for the night and now it is time for rest and relaxation.

Try not to timetable your day so that every minute is accounted for
I used to do this constantly, it was another version of the to-do list, and still find myself reverting back to it sometimes when I am particularly under pressure. If every minute is accounted for, there is no flexibility, no time for a change of plan or something to go awry. Sometimes I find that the universe intervenes, so my perfectly planned day is kyboshed, however, it can turn out to be a better day. If you need to timetable, try to factor in an extra 5–10 minutes between each job; if you finish on time use it for breathing / meditation / daydreaming. If you run late then the pressure is not so great. I am trying to develop my flexibility skills – go with the flow – which is a huge challenge for someone who likes a plan.

Stop the control freak
Why do I find this so hard? For me, this desperate desire to get all my jobs done is a control thing – I'm working on it, and now actively look for ways to lighten my load. When someone asks if they can help in the kitchen, for example, instead of saying 'No I'm fine' (secretly thinking they won't chop the carrots exactly the way I do them) I think, this is a gift, here is someone offering to help me, to lighten my load how could I be considering saying *no*... Control freakish natures stem from fear. Events from my childhood set up the fear story that has run my life so far. That overriding requirement to be responsible for everybody and everything, for heaven's sake I was the child at the age of 8 who was worrying that my father was going to run out of money because

he was buying us ice creams every day on holiday. The problem with fear from childhood is that, as we become adults, fear is a less easy emotion to admit to so it tends to morph into needing to keep control.

Are you a control freak?
Do you like to have a plan for the day? – YES, drives my husband nuts.

Do you have lots of personal rules and routines – YES, I thought that was being disciplined.

Do you 'help' other people? – tricky one this, as the nature of my job is to help but I have learnt that everyone has their own path and I can't be responsible for / control everyone's healing.

Do you dislike depending on others or allowing them to do things for you – getting there, but it still feels uncomfortable.

Do you like to be right – a resounding YES from my family.

Do you like to be organised? – YES to my diary, work and family stuff, absolutely NO to my physical environment, my office is a tip.

How are you at spontaneity? – I like to have a plan – need I say more.

Do you hate being late? – used to, but this one I have got cracked unless of course I am travelling on public transport – the thought alone is enough to get the cortisol buzzing – I have learnt to leave lots of extra time, much to the disgust of my youngest son who is Mr Zen and likes to screech onto the platform with 30 seconds to spare!

Do you correct people when they are wrong – EEK YES, but just in my head – I don't want to lose all of my friends – probably have now!

Realising that, with many of my jobs, if I leave them till tomorrow the sky will not fall in, was a major breakthrough.

Whizzy mind and switching your head off
Just having constant thoughts running through your head is stressful for the body; it maintains that constant scanning for the sabre-toothed tiger. My solution is to chip away at it and do 5 minutes at a time, scheduling in activities that switch my brain off and calm the body – dog walking I thought was a de-stressing activity until one day I went with my husband. We were walking along and he said:
  'Oh, that gate is broken, how long has it been like that?'
  'I don't know' was my reply.
  'But you walk along here every day, how could you not have noticed?'
  That got me thinking, yes, I walked along there every day but I wasn't really there, I was pounding along with my head down 'getting my exercise', but my head was back in the office, composing emails, thinking about clients or planning what to cook for supper. I was completely missing out on 30 minutes of my day, re-living something that I was going to be doing anyway when I got back from the walk – this was insane. I now try to be *present* with my walk, watch the dogs, wonder what they are thinking, concentrate on my footsteps and chat to the trees. I have a favourite beech tree which I hug every day, I close my eyes and just listen, it is amazing how many different sounds there are in a wood. This approach has also paid dividends when I am riding: I try to be with the horse and feel what he is feeling, otherwise I am lost in my head, which he will pick up very quickly and shy at some terrifying clump of dandelions.
  This is mindfulness: it doesn't have to involve weird postures, double-jointed finger poses or increasing your spirituality (although the latter may be a side effect). It just

involves being in the moment, concentrating on what you are doing at that moment in time. Practise developing your senses – sight, sound, taste, touch and smell – if we can create some stillness in our lives, it becomes so much slower. This sounds like a simple concept, but don't be fooled, in reality your 'monkey mind' will rebel and want to get in on the action.

Monkey mind
Monkey mind was a term coined within the Buddhist religion. Buddha said:

'Just as a monkey swinging through the trees grabs one branch and lets it go only to seize another, so too, that which is called thought, mind or consciousness arises and disappears continually both day and night (S.II,95).'

Your monkey mind is like a small child wanting to be the centre of attention, and it does not respond well to being told to be quiet. It likes to focus on the past or the future, because if you are really in the present moment it does not involve thought. For me it is a work in progress – some days better than others. Ensuring that I am focusing on what I am doing at that moment in time is really helpful. With the meditation thing, I find that it is useful to have something to focus on – a body scan works really well for me, this is where someone talks you through the different parts of your body so you pay full attention to each bit (there are loads online, just find one with a voice that you don't find annoying). If not a body scan / guided meditation, focus on the breath, trying to lengthen the out-breath as much as possible or sit in front of a candle and get lost in the flickering flame.

Limbic anchoring
The limbic system is the creator of all of our emotions, and our emotions are based upon past experience, making it very hard to reason with limbic responses. We come back to the

idea that all our responses to life are a choice, although it may not feel like it most of the time. Our experiences as children are the most powerful: our observations of others, in particular how our parents react to life events, teach us how we should also react. In order to retrain our limbic responses, it is important to be aware of our triggers, and this requires a bit of space and self awareness. Very often a few slow breaths before we react can redirect our response to an event, however, if it is a deep-seated learnt response then it may take a little more work. The most valuable thing to create in your head is a safe space, and this safe space acts as an anchor to bring you back down from your heightened stressed state. The safe space needs to involve all of your senses – sight, sound, touch, taste and smell – and every time you go there your body will be relaxed. Initally the safe space needs to be visited in your head on a regular basis to really cement that feeling of security for the mind and the body. My safe space is in a wood where I walk most days; I am sitting with my back against my favourite beech tree, the sun is filtering through the leaves on to my skin and all of the trees around me are standing as sentries to protect me. I can hear all the sounds of the wood, birds chirruping, leaves rustling, the nearby stream, my spaniel Myrtle is sitting quietly beside me (not usual for a spaniel to sit quietly but when I meditate outside, she will always be close, watching me with her wise eyes). The smell of the wood, which changes through the seasons, is very important. Smell is incredibly emotive, the only sense that goes directly to the amygdala, and the amygdala is in charge of what memories we store. Smell is emotive only through association: we can teach our bodies to react to smells in a beneficial way. I suggest that to train your smell response you get some essential oil and carry it with you, a fragrance or mixture of fragrances that you really love (mine is frankincense). Every time you are feeling particularly calm and relaxed have a good sniff. The essential oils particularly associated with calming are lavender, rose, ylang ylang, frankincense, bergamot and chamomile. The association between your calm feeling and the fragrance will become strongly cemented, so if at any point you start to feel anxious a good sniff with some slow deep breaths can help to switch you out of fight / flight. We can also practise this with music: my calming music is *Return to Now: Namaste music* by Buddha's Lounge. I first listened to this during a couple of Relaxation Yoga sessions, which helped to cement in my body that this music was all about feeling relaxed, nurtured and safe. I now listen to it when I am doing relaxing activities to keep it cemented, but if I am feeling wired or anxious about something, I can also put it on to calm me down.

The value of meditation

With the advances of neuro-science we can now track the benefits of what meditation does for the brain – studies show that it can increase the amount of grey matter[79] involved in learning and memory, emotion regulation, speech, decision-making, sense of self and self-control.

It can help to balance blood sugar levels,[80] reduce stress hormones,[81] reduce blood pressure[82] and boost the immune system.[83]

Not bad for just sitting quietly. All of the above health benefits are brilliant, but for me one of the most valuable elements is that I have to sit with myself and pay attention to my thoughts and feelings. This has provided me with much insight as to what is going on, why I am behaving as I am and what I can try and do about it.

Often when I mention meditation to clients, they pull a face and say 'I tried that, I just couldn't do it.' In my experience there is no such thing as not being able to meditate. Admittedly some days are better than others but I think there is a belief that you *have* to enter this zen state of bliss

every time you meditate in order to benefit from it. This
simply is not true. I certainly don't achieve this often, in fact
very rarely; most days my mind is bouncing around all over
the place, but I stick with it, keep letting the thoughts go
and return to focusing on my breathing. I do this every day
for 20 minutes first thing in the morning, before my day
really kicks into action. The major benefit I have noticed is
that I am generally a lot calmer (I think my family would
vouch for this?), I'm not saying I don't have a way to go, but
life is a process. See RESOURCES for meditation help.

Do you need a digital detox?
As well as protecting our body from EMR, a digital detox
can do wonders for the busyness of our minds. A few questions for you:

When you hear the phone go ping etc do you drop
whatever you're doing and check your phone?

Do you feel anxious when you're unable to check your
phone / social media updates?

Do you sleep with your phone?

Do you check your phone before you even get out of
bed?

Have you ever texted or read texts whilst driving?

Do you check your phone to fill the time?

Do you check your phone when you are talking to someone else?

Mobile phone addiction is a recognised phenomenon:
every time we look at them we get a small dopamine rush.
Dopamine is the reward neurotransmitter that is produced
when we eat sugar or take drugs like heroin. It makes us feel
good, but with feel-good hormones there has to be a balance
and there will always be a slight down afterwards. This drives
us back to more phone time to get our dopamine 'hit'. The

trouble is that bodies require more and more dopamine to get the same level of positive emotion so we end up being more and more glued to our phones.

Some ideas that might help are:

Get the phone out of the bedroom and try to not let it be the first thing that you look at when you come downstairs – at least make a cup of (herbal) tea first. If you meditate in the morning, I urge you not to look at your phone before you do this as it just gives more for the monkey mind to work on when you are trying to be still.

Set a time slot / slots in the day when you will not check any electronic device. Be very firm about your intention – the average person checks 150 times a day. What are we checking for? Most of the time the information coming in is a waste of our time. Put your phone out of sight and on silent so it is not so tempting.

Dsisconnecting, this really helps to reduce that feeling of overload. Set a challenge – how long can your tech-free time last?

Do not even attempt to look at your phone when you are conversing with another human being, or animal for that matter.

If you are going out, ask the question: do I really need to take my phone?

Have tech-free zones in the house – for starters the place where you come together to eat and talk to each other.

When you exercise, make it a phone-free zone. It is very tempting to do another job when you take exercise. The sky will not fall in if you are out of the loop for 30–60 minutes and if that little voice pipes up saying but there might be an EMERGENCY, kick it into touch: how many true emergencies can we realistically expect in life?

Be aware of why you are checking your phone – is it because there is nothing else to do, perhaps you are walking along a street or waiting for an appointment or sitting in a traffic jam. Check your phone because you need to, not because there is a gap in your life.

Creating balance

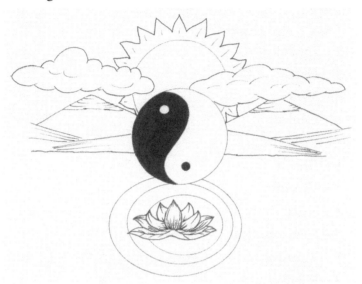

Yin and yang – although these two energies are total opposites, they are also completely interdependent – one cannot exist without the other. The light part of the symbol represents yang energy and the dark side the yin energy. It is vital for vibrant health that both of these energies are in balance. Twenty-first-century living, with its emphasis on speed and achievement, tends to be rather yang dominated. The properties of yang are:

- Masculine
- Light
- Sun
- Heat
- Active
- Strong
- Conqueror

- Interventionist
- Open
- Movement
- Day

The yin represents:
- Feminine
- Dark
- Moon
- Coolness
- Reflective
- Gentle
- Conquered
- Subtle
- Compassionate
- Inclusive
- Stillness
- Night

It is important for men as well as women to nurture their yin side.

For me, because I was, and often still am, running stress, my go-to phrase can be 'I just haven't got time' – even for nice things, which tend to be the more yin-nurturing activities. These are:

- Resting
- Playing
- Relaxing
- Spending time in mother nature
- Communicating in person rather than electronically

I now have to stop myself when that phrase pops up and take a moment to think about whether I have enough balance. What yin-nourishing activities are there in my day?

The balance of yin and yang permeates every moment of our existence.

The balance between:

Waking and Sleeping – to support yin we need to ensure we are getting enough sleep.

Work and Play / Rest.

What we are eating can also affect the yin / yang balance. In order to support yin, below are a few foods that are useful to incorporate into our diet, they are foods that are more 'cooling', rather than the yang foods which tend to make us overheat, like coffee, alcohol and sugar.

- Avocado
- Egg
- Lemon
- Nettle
- Sesame
- Spinach
- Sweet potato
- Tomato
- Seaweed
- Pear
- Crab
- Apple
- Malt
- Asparagus
- Pomegranate
- String beans

The importance of laughter, humour and positivity

'If you have good thoughts they will shine out of your face
like sunbeams and you will always look lovely.' — Roald Dahl

Laughter and humour are fabulous de-stressors[84] and if you
lose these from your life it is a sure sign that your zen mission is not going to plan.

Laughter:
- Stimulates all the main organs
- Increases the amount of oxygen we inhale
- Relaxes the muscles
- Boosts the immune system
- Relieves pain
- Increases ability to cope with stressful situations

How to increase humour and laughter
- Set an intention at the beginning of the day to laugh
  more or even just smile more
- Watch funny films or read funny books
- Put funny sayings or cartoons around the place
- Google funny clips
- Be more silly – play silly games
- Hang out with funny people
- Sign up for laughter yoga

If you are a long-term stress-head who has been running
fight / flight for decades, be gentle with yourself: your body
is doing its best to keep you safe but just doesn't realise the
majority of the time it *is* safe. If we think of our adrenals as
a bank account, many are overdrawn; try to think of daily
things to top up our account. The calming process doesn't

happen overnight, stick with it, check in with your body regularly, reassure it that no danger lurks in the shadows. You will slowly start to realise that your reactions to things are calmer, time seems to go a bit more slowly and that you become more observant about your surroundings because you are living in the moment, not in the past or in the future.

'We may not be responsible for the world that created our minds, but we can take responsibility for the mind with which we create our world.'

— Gabor Mate

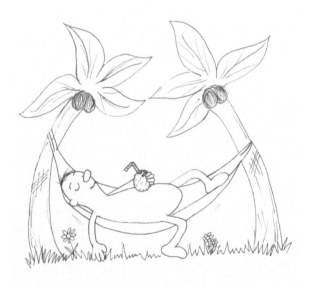

9

SUGAR

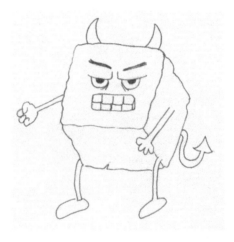

In my opinion, sugar in excess is the single most damaging natural food that we can put into our bodies. Obesity levels are soaring and the main culprit is sugar consumption. According to Public Health England, ⅔ of adults, ⅓ of 11–15-year-olds and ¼ of 2–10-year-olds fall into the overweight or obese category. Since 2006, tooth extractions on children aged 4 and under have risen by 25%. Sugar is causing major damage to the health and wellbeing of all who consume it in excess.

As I have said, sugar acts like a drug. One of my lecturers stated that if sugar came on the market now it would be on prescription only, it is so damaging and so addictive. Sugar has been proven to be as addictive as cocaine, after all it is derived from plants and refined into pure white crystals! The Dutch Health Minister in 2013, Paul van der Velpen (cannabis is legal in the Netherlands), was trying to get sugar reclassified as a drug as it interferes with the body's appetite messages and leads to an insatiable urge to continue eating.

'Just like alcohol and tobacco, sugar is actually a drug. There is an important role for government. The use of sugar should be discouraged. And users should be made aware of the dangers.'[85]

In Dutch schools they have banned fruit juice. Unfortunately, in the UK no one in our government is courageous enough to attempt this, despite Jamie Oliver's valiant efforts. Some half-hearted attempts have been made to reduce sugar in fizzy drinks, but this is a drop in the ocean.

WHAT HAPPENS WHEN WE EAT SUGAR

From birth, as a survival mechanism, we have a sweet tooth – those that could consume more fast-release energy were more likely to survive. No wonder it is such a hard habit to kick. When we eat sugar, and it doesn't just have to be the white grainy stuff – we shouldn't kid ourselves – honey, molasses, agave nectar, maple syrup, dates, all these supposedly 'healthy' sugars produce an insulin response, in order to reduce blood sugar levels. Unfortunately, it is not just the sweet stuff that raises blood sugar: if you eat a slice of white bread it is equivalent to eating 1.3gms of sugar, an average baked potato is equivalent to 3gms of sugar … so you see how easy it is to rack up the amount of sugar you are consuming, even if you do not have a sweet tooth. Refined carbohydrates, in fact all carbohydrates, are a source of sugar to a greater or lesser degree.

At the beginning of the 20th century, the average sugar consumption was 1lb a week, now it is 6lbs. That is 3 bags of sugar a week, and not surprisingly there has got to be some fallout: our bodies simply cannot cope with this quantity.

When we eat sugar, it raises our blood sugar levels, excess sugar is bad news in the bloodstream – if it hangs around, it tends to stick to things. Firstly, to the blood vessels' walls (heart disease), and secondly to the white blood cells which prevents them from fighting infections, or seeking out and destroying cancer cells. It also sticks to our red blood cells and reduces their ability to carry oxygen round the body. The HbA1c test is a useful blood test to show how much this has been happening – it will give you a reading of how much the haemoglobin (red blood cells) have been glycated (sugar molecule stuck to it) over the previous 3 months, so there is no good in eating virtuously the week before your test!

It is important that the body deals with this sugar as quickly as possible, so insulin is produced, which travels around in the bloodstream asking the cells to take up the excess sugar. If your blood sugar levels have been quite high, a large amount of insulin is produced. Now insulin is a powerful hormone and will reduce your blood sugar levels efficiently but as blood sugar levels start to slump so can we. Low and high blood sugar can be equally stressful for the body. The brain is very sensitive to low blood sugar and will send out messages saying 'We are in a life-threatening situation here – I NEED MORE SUGAR.' This is the point where we have that mid-morning or mid-afternoon energy slump, where it feels like a coffee and biscuit, piece of chocolate, muffin etc are absolutely essential to prevent us from:

- biting the head off a colleague / family member – low blood sugar can make you extremely irritable
- getting the shakes – this is your nervous system being stimulated
- putting our heads down on the desk and having a little snooze
- making a bad decision due to confusion
- getting heart palpitations

- feeling light-headed / dizzy

Sugary snacks, refined carbohydrates and stimulants, e.g. coffee, tea and alcohol, will all raise blood sugar levels. The stimulants do this because (although we may have a coffee / tea without sugar) they prepare the body for action and of course this means we need sugar in the bloodstream. A blood sugar spike usually results in an ensuing slump. This rollercoaster of blood sugar levels peaking and troughing is what I see in about 80% of my clients, and it causes untold damage in the body. If this situation continues, with insulin constantly being produced to deal with high blood sugar levels, the cells start to become resistant to the insulin message and will not take up any more sugar from the bloodstream.

This is called insulin resistance, and is a sign that the body is heading towards becoming diabetic.

Signs and symptoms of insulin resistance are:
Weight gain around the middle – check hip to waist ratio, which is the waist measurement divided by the hip measurement. For optimal health women's should be less than 0.8 and for men it should be less than 0.95.

Fatigue after carbohydrate meals.

Sugar cravings – because insulin is not able to get sugar into the cells they are actually starving for sugar.

Night sweats, irritability, palpitations, dizziness, fatigue relieved by eating. This is because the insulin is not working in getting the sugar into the cells for their proper function.

Chronic fungal infections – thrush (vaginal or oral), fungal toenails, athlete's foot. Sugar feeds yeast.

Skin tags, these are little growths that usually are found where the skin forms creases e.g. neck, armpit, groin; they can also appear on the eyelids. Insulin is a growth hormone – an excess of it encourages excess growth.

Excess sugar in the bloodstream is sent to the liver where it is converted to fat and the fat is deposited around the middle so it is near to the liver to break down if needed at a future date. As we know visceral fat causes all sorts of problems of its own, disrupting appetite and promoting inflammation. One hormone that is key in disrupting our appetite is leptin. Leptin in appropriate amounts is a really helpful hormone, as it serves to reduce our appetite by making us feel full. This hormone tells our brain that we have enough fat stored and that we don't need to eat any more calories. This hormone is brilliant for helping us to lose weight if there is not too much of it around, but excess fat cells produce excess leptin, and like with insulin our cells become resistant to the leptin message. If this message does not get through, our brain thinks that we don't have enough fat stored and that we are starving, hence will ramp up our appetite and reduce our energy expenditure – disaster when we are trying to lose weight.

THE KEY TO WEIGHT-LOSS IS TO EAT A DIET THAT REQUIRES A MINIMAL INSULIN RESPONSE AND REDUCES OUR LEPTIN LEVELS

Insulin resistance, prediabetes and Type 2 diabetes are all completely reversible conditions: you need to get the cells responding to insulin again, it takes a bit of homework, but it is totally achievable. One of the most effective ways for people to lose weight is to cut out all carbs and sugar – this is effectively the paleo way of eating, what we ate when we were living in caves, i.e. meat, fish, eggs, nuts, seeds, fruit, vegetables and good quantities of fat. I am not an advocate of a high-protein paleo diet, it is important to balance the protein with lots of plant matter – this does not include lots of beans and pulses as they are quite high in carbohydrate. My plate would be about ¼–⅓ protein and the rest would be vegetables (that doesn't include potatoes, but sweet ones are OK). It is also important to not go mad on the fruit – 2 portions a day maximum, and always remember to eat your fruit don't drink it. When we extract the juice from fruit, we are taking out all the sugary bits to consume and removing all the fibre, which slows down the sugar release into the bloodstream.

Eating this way does not require such an insulin response (fat cells only proliferate and thrive in the presence of insulin), our blood sugar levels will be kept much more even, not swinging up and down, and we find that we are not so hungry.

To help reduce leptin levels, reduce the carbs and increase fibre and protein. It is also important to make sure that you are getting enough exercise and sleep.

DON'T BE TEMPTED TO RESORT TO SWEETENERS

The following are a few common ways that food manufacturers sweeten things by not actually using sugar so that they can claim their product is low sugar.

Aspartame – this is the most toxic of the sweeteners: it contains methanol molecules, which are converted by an enzyme called alcohol dehydrogenase into formaldehyde. There are a multitude of metabolic and neurological side effects associated with this substance, in particular it is found to mess about with the antioxidant status in the brain,[86] other issues range from birth defects, cancer and diabetes to seizures and depression.

Saccharin has been linked to bladder cancer in rats; research into what it does to humans came up with the reassurance that it was 'unlikely' to cause cancer in humans.

Sucralose – this is sucrose that has had a chlorine molecule added to it. This means that you don't absorb it but the breakdown products are carcinogenic. Sucralose can reduce your good gut bacteria and affect the liver enzymes that help you detox and process medications.[87]

Sorbitol – this is particularly dangerous for diabetics as they have an increased amount of the enzyme aldose reductase in their system. This enzyme converts glucose to sorbitol which means that diabetics very quickly get toxic levels of sorbitol in the bloodstream, leading to damage to nerves, blood vessels, eyes and kidneys.

Acesulfame K – found to create DNA damage in mice; again, it may not be harmful to humans but I don't want to take that chance.

If you are going to eat sugar then make sure it is a sugar that is non-toxic, and one that the body can recognise, not some weird Frankenstein sugar cooked up in a laboratory.

Sweeteners generally affect our appetite control centre and metabolism. They have been proven to stimulate our appetite and carbohydrate cravings and increase our fat storage. As sweeteners are not real sugar the body does not register them as such, so it means that it cannot accurately calculate the amount of calories that we have consumed and give us the message that we are satisfied. The sweet taste stimulates our appetite but there are no calories to follow, so we still feel hungry.

What we need to understand about the sweet taste is that it signals to our body that it is about to receive a big dose of calories, therefore it prepares for those calories by producing extra insulin, and we know that excess insulin causes more fat storage.

If you are thoroughly depressed by the thought of having to cut out sugar, there is a small glimmer of hope in the form of xylitol. Xylitol is a sugar that despite its very chemical-sounding name is natural and extracted from birch trees and other hardwoods. It is being promoted by the medical world for various reasons, firstly it is very low GI (glycemic index) so it does not spike blood sugar levels and is more suitable for diabetics. Secondly, dentists are promoting it because unlike sugar it is not converted into acids in the mouth which cause tooth decay. At the moment there is no evidence to show that xylitol causes problems in the body, although if you eat large amounts you can get water retention in the gut, which can cause diarrhoea, and if you have imbalanced gut bacteria it can make you rather windy. My gut feeling about xylitol is that we need to be wary and not overdo it with this product. I have come to the conclusion that there is no free lunch when it comes to sugar and consuming even xylitol does not train our taste buds to crave less of the sweet stuff. If we take the sweet taste out of our diet, which will help to balance the gut bacteria, we (and our gut bacteria) will then no longer be hunting around for the little sweet something.

A word about agave nectar, which is very high in fructose, i.e. fruit sugar.

BUT FRUIT SUGAR IS HEALTHY ISN'T IT?

Fruit contains sugar and when we consume it, as a hangover from our hunter-gatherer days, it signals to the body that it is summer / autumn time. In the past this was a time when we needed to stockpile a bit of extra girth to get us through the freezing days of winter. Our bodies have not evolved fast enough for this mechanism to be upgraded, so when we eat any type of sugar, even when it is from fruit, a message tells the body that we need to store fat.

The other problem with fruit sugar is that it has a high content of fructose, which is actually toxic to the liver.[88] High-fructose corn syrup, a cheap way of sweetening foods, is being held responsible for much of the obesity and obesity-related conditions of today. Dr Robert Lustig, author of *Fat Chance: The Bitter Truth about Sugar*, describes it as a 'chronic, dose-dependent liver toxin'. The difference between glucose and fructose is that fructose cannot be used by cells for energy, it has to be metabolised in the liver first. The end result of metabolising fructose in the liver is that it produces excess triglycerides (involved in the development of heart disease) and excess free radicals. Fructose also messes about with the mechanisms that make us feel full and satisfied, so we are far more likely to eat more of something sweetened with fructose than we are if it is sweetened with glucose.

A WORD ABOUT ALCOHOL

Just so we are under no illusions – alcohol is sugar, and here is a general guideline, although it does depend upon the brand.

1 pint of beer – approx 2 teaspoons

1 gin and tonic – approx 3 teaspoons of sugar – mostly due to the tonic

1 glass of wine – approx 1 teaspoon

HOW CAN WE HELP TO BALANCE OUR BLOOD SUGAR

As protein is harder to break down than carbohydrate, this slows down the digestion process, meaning that the sugar release will be more gradual, lessening the likelihood of a blood sugar spike.

Eating protein with every meal / snack helps to keep energy levels more constant, which in turn helps to keep our mood more even because fluctuating blood sugar levels can affect production of brain chemicals.[89]

Another important point to remember at this juncture is that high stress levels unbalance our blood sugar. One of my clients who was reversing her Type 2 diabetes, and so recording her blood sugar levels regularly, could very accurately track her stress levels by what her blood sugar levels were doing. Once her levels were under control and she was off her medication, the spikes were never due to what she was eating, it was her fight / flight response being triggered. Weight-loss is not just about what we are consuming: our stress levels can play a big role.

FASTING AND ITS BENEFITS

For me the idea of fasting is an abhorrent one – food is one of the highlights of my day, and here we are talking about *missing* meals! However, in the interests of my own health I decided to give it a try and it is really not that bad once you get into the swing of it. I suggest that you start with trying the intermittent version.

Once you have stabilised your blood sugar levels, e.g. you don't get dizzy, irritable, shaky if you don't eat regularly, and you still have weight to lose you can then look at intermittent fasting: this is eating all of your meals within 8 hours (or less) of a 24-hour period. Basically, missing breakfast or having a late breakfast and early supper is usually the easiest way to do this. If you have very disordered blood sugar balance you may have to ease yourself into this process and have a couple of spoonfuls of coconut oil at breakfast time. This will give your body some fuel but it will not stimulate an insulin response.

Facts about fasting

Three meals a day is a modern convention – research has shown that a body fares much better if it gets all of its fuel within an 8-hour window, or even less. Keeping the body in a fasting state is most beneficial.

Fasting is an integral part of many religions – Muhammed, Buddha and Jesus all made fasting a part of their religious practice.

As Rumi said, 'Fasting is the first principle of medicine; fast and see the strength of the spirit reveal itself.'

Fasting teaches the body to balance its own blood sugar.

Fasting helps to reduce sugar cravings – as your body starts to balance its blood sugar levels it won't have the dips and so won't need sugar to resolve this.

Fasting improves your gut bacteria; if you have imbalanced gut bacteria you will be feeding the pathogenic ones less.

If you have become insulin resistant – see signs and symptoms above – fasting is the best way to increase the sensitivity of your cells to insulin again.

Fasting gives your whole system a rest, in particular the whole digestive tract, the liver and the kidneys.

The immune system gets a rest as it is not constantly having to investigate any bits of food that might leak through the gut wall.

Fasting gives the body a chance to have a bit of a spring clean. When it is not having to put time and energy into digesting, one of the processes that it triggers is autophagy (effectively self digestion): the body will clear out any damaged components within the cell, and if the cell is damaged enough it will digest the whole thing – this includes cancerous cells.

Fasting teaches the body to start using fat as a fuel with the inevitable result of weight-loss.

Fasting can help brain function as it boosts the amount of BDNF (brain-derived neurotrophic factor) that we produce. I have heard BDNF described as 'Miracle Grow' for our brains, it activates brain stem cells to grow into new brain cells or neurons. It is a myth that we cannot grow new brain cells.

Fasting helps you live longer – the very process of digestion produces free radicals. As free radicals are our main cause of ageing, eating less increases longevity. Studies done with animals including rats, mice, worms, flies, fish and spiders on a calorie-restricted diet show up to a 50% increase in longevity.[90]

Fasting inhibits the mTOR pathway. This is a pathway that regulates cell growth and proliferation, and by inhibiting this pathway it gets the cell to upregulate the amount of maintenance and repair done.

THE IMPORTANCE OF MITOCHONDRIA

Fasting helps the health of our mitochondria. Mitochondria are minute organelles, of which there are approximately 10 million billion in an adult body, accounting for about 10% of body weight. It is believed that if it weren't for these tiny organelles, we may not have developed beyond a primitive life form.

Mitochondria are responsible for producing energy, and if they are not functioning properly everything is on go-slow *and I mean everything*, from muscle contraction to digestion to thought processes to hormone production.

Mitochondrial function can be affected by:

Nutritional deficiencies – B vitamins, magnesium and essential fat, to name a few, are all vital for the efficient running of these powerhouses.

Toxins – pollution, chemicals in food, toxic toiletries, prescription medication etc.

Chronic viral or bacterial infection.

High levels of oxidation / free radicals in the body.

High levels of inflammation.

Stress.

If we are feeling exhausted, it might seem to make sense that our body needs more fuel but excessive levels of food mean that the body generates excess free radicals and this can hamper the function of the mitochondria.

Fasting a few hours before we go to bed is most beneficial because this is when our body is at its lowest metabolic rate so we are not consuming calories that we don't need. I find that if I go to bed slightly hungry, I will have a much better quality of sleep, and wake feeling more refreshed. However,

I will caveat that with the fact that I have spent some time getting my blood sugar control to work efficiently. If the body is not having to digest it can concentrate on all the other important functions that occur during sleep.

A SHORT WORD ABOUT ENERGY PRODUCTION AND CHRONIC FATIGUE SYNDROME

Chronic Fatigue Syndrome is something that I am seeing more and more in my practice. Poor functioning mitochondria usually have a large part to play. This is a complex and very distressing disease that, in particular, I have seen kybosh the lives of young people. If you are in this situation or have a loved one who is, then I recommend that you start with reading Dr Sarah Myhill's book *Chronic Fatigue Syndrome – 'It's mitochondria, not hypochondria.'* This will help you to understand what is going on in the body on a physical basis and help redress imbalances. In addition, however, with this issue there is *always* an emotional element, and for this I urge you to get in touch with the Optimum Health Clinic in London. This clinic specialises in Chronic Fatigue / ME / fibromyalgia, and most of the practitioners have suffered from these conditions and recovered, so they really know what they are talking about. They can help you to understand your type of character and modes of operating, which are usually exacerbating the situation, along with any traumas that may be running the system and putting your body into fight / flight more than it should be.

MY TOP TIP FOR GETTING OFF THE SUGAR

When we eat sugar, it releases opioids and dopamine into the system: these are the same substances that flood a body when taking cocaine, so no wonder it is so hard to kick the sugar habit. If you are a real sugar junky, my advice is to go cold turkey. If I had a cocaine addict in front of me, I would not be advising them to just cut down a bit – that would be ludicrous. Well, in the same way it makes life very challenging if we just cut down a bit on the sugar. That little bit of the sweet stuff has us just wanting more, and before we know it that chocolate bar / packet of biscuits is finished. It is far easier to cut it out completely – try it for two to three weeks and you will be amazed at how quickly the sugar cravings disappear. You will also find that your taste for sweet things reduces. Getting a sugar habit under control is, from a dietary point of view, the most beneficial thing that we can achieve for our long-term health.

10

SLEEP

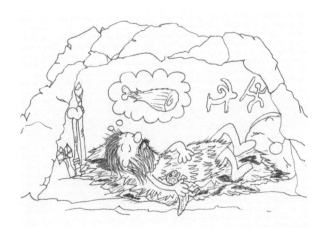

In the words of sleep scientist Cheri Mah, 'An optimal sleep environment is a cave – dark, quiet, cool, comfortable.'

Sleep is such an undervalued activity, and unfortunately operating on a lack of it seems to be a badge of honour. People like Margaret Thatcher (famed for her four hours a night) and Ronald Reagan were admired for their seeming lack of sleep requirement. Could the fact that both ended up with dementia be connected – who knows?

On a good regime, we spend approximately one third of our lives asleep; however, before the invention of artificial light, people tended to have more like 10 hours a night. All other animals regulate their diurnal patterns with light and dark but human beings have stopped doing that. It is recommended that we get 8 hours sleep, but I don't have many clients that are achieving this. Personally, I get about 7½; I get up at 6am which means that I have to be quite disciplined about going to bed at a decent time. I don't need to wake up to an alarm and feel refreshed when I wake, this is my benchmark of whether I am getting enough sleep. I have realised (as I don't drink much alcohol) that most of my hangovers, when I have them, are lack of sleep.

Sleep is a hugely important part of optimal health and something that often seems to go haywire if we are overly stressed. The adrenals play a very important part in keeping us asleep. As our blood sugar levels drop when we are sleeping it is vital that our cortisol levels are gently rising through the night to prevent blood sugar from dropping too low. If our adrenals are overworked and they do not produce enough cortisol, then blood sugar levels can drop enough to alert the brain. The brain is very sensitive to levels of sugar and will have a bit of a panic in the night, sending emergency messages to the adrenals to produce cortisol and sometimes a bit of adrenalin if things are feeling really life-threatening. These stress hormones can be enough to wake us up – sometimes with a pounding heart – then that old monkey mind will kick in and you lie there for hours thinking about the next day and how much there is to do and how tired you are going to be in the morning. Before we look at ways to help with sleep I would just like to run through how important it is.

Whilst sleeping we are:

Processing emotions – if people are having ongoing disturbing dreams / nightmares this indicates that there is unprocessed emotion that the brain can't 'put to bed'. If this is your experience I suggest that some EMDR therapy may well help with this – see page 201. Sleep can also be extremely useful for resolving knotty problems:

how many times do you go to sleep with a problem and it seems to be resolved in the morning?

'It is a common experience that a problem difficult at night is resolved in the morning after the committee of sleep has worked on it.' — John Steinbeck

Improving our memories.

Consolidating newly acquired skills.

Reducing inflammation – people who sleep more have lower levels of C-Reactive Protein[91] (an indicator of inflammation).

Cleaning the brain – it has been discovered that when we are asleep our brain cells shrink a bit, which leaves a vacuum. This vacuum is filled with cerebrospinal fluid which rushes in and around the neurons, removing waste and proteins like beta-amyloid. Beta-amyloid can accumulate into plaques and contribute to Alzheimer's and dementia. This is known as the 'glymphatic system'. Less sleep means less time for cleaning.

Slowing down and regulating our heart rate and blood pressure.

Helping to regulate our appetite – sleep suppresses the hormone ghrelin, which makes you hungry. If we are tired and sleepy, production of ghrelin is increased. Sleep has been proven to be part of an effective weight-loss strategy.

Repair and regeneration of tissue; this involves the immune system which has been shown to be impaired with sleep restriction.[92]

Detoxing – as well as cleaning the brain, this is when the liver is most active. In traditional Chinese medicine, it is shown that each of the main organs in the body has a time slot within our 24-hour cycle, when it becomes more active. The liver time is between 1–3am, so if you find that you are consistently waking up at this time, it might be your liver trying to tell you something (it can also be adrenals).

I list below the organs, their times and associated emotions – if we have something that is out of balance or a particular time of day when we always feel sluggish it might be worth looking into the function of that organ and whether it needs some support.

Liver 1–3am – Anger

Lungs 3–5am – Grief

Large Intestines 5–7am – Sadness

Stomach 7–9am – Fear

Spleen and Pancreas 9–11am – Self-esteem

Heart and Mind 11–1pm – Ruler of all emotions

Small Intestine 1–3pm – Mental deficiency – forgetfulness, indecision

Bladder 3–5pm – Resisting change and Negativity

Kidneys 5–7pm – Insecurity and Fear

Pericardium (protective sac around our heart) 7–9pm – Difficulty expressing emotions

Triple Warmer Meridian (the meridian responsible for production and circulation of protective and nourishing energy) 9–11pm – Joy

Gall Bladder 11–1am – Indecision and timidity

CIRCADIAN RHYTHM

Our body has its own 24-hour clock – the circadian rhythm – and many processes are governed by this. Processes such as sleeping and waking, blood pressure control, eating, reactivity of our immune system (people with allergies like hay fever are often worse in the morning), and ability to process medications. Much of our hormone production is controlled by the circadian rhythm and our friend cortisol is very much included in this. If our cortisol rhythm is working correctly then levels will be high in the morning, which gets us bouncing out of bed, and they will lessen over the day so that by bedtime our body knows that it is time to wind down and go to sleep. They will then slowly rise through the night in order to stop our blood sugar levels from dropping too low. Many of my clients have disordered sleep because their fight / flight is switched on and there is too much cortisol produced through the day, meaning levels are too high at bedtime. This makes it very hard to get off to sleep. Alternatively, if the high cortisol situation has gone on for a while the adrenals are exhausted so cortisol levels are low and people drop off as soon as their head hits the pillow but there is not enough production of cortisol through the night to keep blood sugar levels even. If the adrenals are overworked, and our cortisol levels are flatlining it means that we will be hitting the snooze button a lot and dragging ourselves out of bed. If we have also had a restless night and spent some of it lying awake with our mind whizzing this is compounded. A good test for me as to whether I am getting enough good-quality sleep is if I wake up naturally – no alarm clock. Some clients say 'I can't do that, I'd sleep all day.' I think that may be your answer, your body needs more rest. As adults we should all be getting between 7–8 hours sleep (teenagers often need a lot more). The problem is there are so many more interesting things to do in the evening than going to bed – just another episode of that box set, getting lost in the world of internet / social media, just winding down from the day if you have been at it till 9–10pm.

Not only has screentime provided us with an excuse not to go to bed but exposure to blue light emitted from any computers, smart phones, iPads etc in the evening disrupts our circadian rhythm. It is important that we do have exposure to blue light (this can be provided by the sun but it should come, ideally, in the morning hours only). Blue light is detected by the pineal gland in the brain, which then suppresses levels of melatonin – 'the hormone of darkness'. Melatonin's prime function is to help us drop off and stay asleep. Getting outside, preferably earlier in the day, is a really good way to help regulate our rhythm and help us to sleep.

FUNCTIONS OF MELATONIN

Helps regulate the sleep–wake cycle by causing drowsiness and lowering the body temperature.

Acts as an antioxidant by scavenging those free radicals, especially in the brain, and because of this function it has been shown not only to act against cancer cells, but also help reduce inflammation and ageing. As we get older many people get brown spots on the backs of their hands – an accumulation of a substance called lipofuscin and indicates increased levels of oxidation in the body. Adequate sleep can be a simple way to reduce age spots.

Helps support the immune system – melatonin talks to the immune system, in particular white blood cells involved in the body's ability to recognise self and non-self – so important when it comes to autoimmune diseases.

I know how unrealistic it is to expect everyone to switch off the screens in the evening, although I do suggest that you try to have a period of downtime for your brain before bed. There are apps that you can download onto computers and phones etc that block the blue light emissions, and there are also amber glasses (this is my approach: my children say they look very fetching and add to my general weirdness) that block blue light. I also wear them watching TV, as televisions also emit blue light.

Whilst we are on the subject of TV, and sleep, it is important to remember that the body cannot differentiate between what it is watching and reality. If you are watching a heart-pumping thriller, your body will be in fight / flight mode ready to keep you safe. This also goes for stressful thoughts: if you are the sort of person that catastrophises and goes off on a journey in your head about the worst-case scenario, your body will think that is really happening. If you are struggling with insomnia may I suggest that you are careful about what you go to bed on, ideally not the news – so depressing and often full of traumatic violent images. If you are hooked on thrillers make a conscious effort to not watch them immediately before going to bed, and be aware of what your body is doing whilst watching them. I find that often I hold my breath if I watch anything remotely suspenseful. Try to make sure that you are breathing slowly and steadily, lengthen the out-breath and talk to your body, reassuring it that this is not reality. If your fight / flight mechanism has got to the stage where it is constantly on surveillance for danger and reacts at the drop of a hat, I suggest that you don't watch these programmes at all. Look for gentle comedy or anything with David Attenborough in it. Apart from the fact that stressful TV switches your fight / flight on there is another reason.

RETICULAR ACTIVATING SYSTEM (RAS)

This is the brain's attention centre, to which all of our senses apart from smell are wired. We are constantly being bombarded with information and the RAS helps to filter out what is important and allows this through into our consciousness. In a bid to make sense of the world, it is constantly scanning for familiarity in order to make connections. If we go to bed on negative, stressful thoughts, then this is what the RAS will be scanning for overnight – not great for a restful, fulfilling night's sleep. The same goes for when we are awake: if we focus on the negative then this is what the RAS will filter into our consciousness. I try to have a minute when I climb into bed thinking about all the good things that have happened that day, no matter how tough the day has been there is always something that I can find to be grateful for.

MAKE YOUR BODY FEEL SAFE AND SECURE

A body that feels safe will relax into good-quality sleep, but if it has been used to scanning all day for the sabre-toothed tiger it is not suddenly going to relax into 8 hours of solid zonked-out sleep, it is just not safe to do so. It can be very helpful to have at least an hour or two when we really concentrate on reassuring the body and helping it to wind down – having a long soak in a bath with Epsom salts, playing some chill out music, reading a calm / funny book or listening to the Calm app (which has some great bedtime stories read by celebrities to lull you off to sleep – they really do work).

Experiment with finding what helps to make your body feel safe so that it can relax into good-quality restorative and healing sleep.

11

SPIRIT

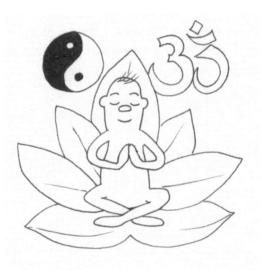

We are incredibly sensitive beings and it does not take much to knock our sense of self. However, I accept that these hardships and adverse experiences are part of our 'development programme'. I hesitate to use the words spiritual development, as this can be off-putting for many.

My wise son once commented, 'Mum, life doesn't happen to you, it happens for you.'

I believe that we are put on this earth to learn lessons and, as I look around me, some of the lessons at earth school are phenomenally tough. I see good honest souls being battered by life events and it is hard to understand what is going on. The wonderful work of Caroline Myss has helped me to try and make sense of this, and I would recommend any of her books or courses.

Our lessons can begin very early, even in the womb. Childhood can be a particularly steep learning curve, but the learning still seems to keep on coming throughout life. Sometimes I long to get off the hamster wheel for a bit of a break, but that is not the way that our 'development' seems to work. Not only do we have our present experiences to deal with but past generations can also pass down their trauma and baggage.

TRANSGENERATIONAL DAMAGE

There are a number of ways transgenerational damage can occur. There is damage that occurs from children observing the behaviour of those around them or experiences in the womb, there is damage that occurs through physical / emotional trauma that is passed down on the genes, and there is also toxic damage, where a child in utero is exposed to a cocktail of toxins.

Let's take the first type – learnt behaviour damage: the behaviour of our parents, care givers, siblings etc teaches us how to navigate and survive in the world, in a bid to try and reduce our exposure to any amount of emotional and physical pain. The strategies that we develop as a child to avoid pain, can be most unhelpful as we grow up.

Let me tell you a story.

Once upon a time there was a little girl called Eleanor; she grew up with doting parents who gave her safe secure boundaries and she was regularly given messages that she was valued and loved. At the age of 3 her father went off to war and a year later the telegram came through to say that he had been killed in action. Her mother was completely devastated by her husband's death and a year later succumbed to tuberculosis. Eleanor, now an orphan, was reluctantly taken in by an aunt who had never married. This aunt was a real character, the life and soul of the party, and it had not been in her game plan to be saddled with a rather quiet and gentle 5-year-old. Eleanor was dragged from pillar to post being shown off at parties like a pet, and she learnt fairly quickly that to get on in the world she had to perform and entertain, otherwise she was discarded as an inconvenience. She grew up being a bright and beautiful butterfly flitting around in society gaining admiration wherever she went in order to salve the deep hurt of abandonment from her childhood. Not surprisingly, when it came to looking for a husband, she looked for a father figure, somebody to fill that hole in her development and her heart. David seemed to fit the bill – strong, serious, steady – and he was blown away by this bright, fragile beauty, somebody to own and protect. His own childhood had also been challenging: a very austere father with a hot temper and a quick hand. David was constantly trying to please and impress him but his achievements were never acknowledged and he grew up feeling a failure despite his accomplishments. In order to cope with the hurt, he learnt that dominating people gave him a sense of control, but underneath there was a little boy constantly seeking approval. If he didn't get it, his hurt quickly turned into anger.

Eleanor and David married quickly and settled down. Soon Eleanor was pregnant and had her first daughter, Sarah, the first of five. Money was short so there was little help and support for Eleanor as she went from one pregnancy to the next. No longer able to be the sparkling socialite to top up her self-esteem, Eleanor descended into depression. She did not have the capacity to love and nurture her own children to make them feel secure and loved, due to her own experiences of abandonment. The eldest child, Sarah, became surrogate mother to the younger ones, in addition to trying to help keep the peace between her increasingly unhappy parents, but Sarah at the age of 10 was poorly equipped with the emotional intelligence to be able to navigate this mine-field of demands and challenging emotions.

In time Sarah grew up, got married and had her own children ... and so many patterns were repeated, in particular perfectionism, people-pleasing, an inability to relax and 'be rather than do'. This trait was then passed on to her own daughter and on down the generations with varying neg-ative effects on health and behaviour. Interestingly, the fe-male members of the family all developed thyroid issues – in the throat area. Was this to do with them feeling unable to communicate their needs and authentic selves?

***

This is a very simplistic view of transgenerational damage, and there are a multitude of different combinations that can shape us and affect our offspring, be they male or female.

The work of Bruce Lipton explores the idea that, up until the age of seven, we are in download mode. This means that we haven't developed the emotional intelligence to process an experience effectively, and then file it properly in the brain. These early experiences are put onto our hard drive, and this is what we end up running our lives by. It is interesting to note a line attributed to St Francis Xavier (1506–1552): 'Give me the child until he is seven and I'll show you the man.' It was recognised then that belief sys-tems can be set for life in young children. If we are told as a child that 'You *are* very naughty,' as opposed to 'What you *did* was very naughty', then this goes on to the hard drive as 'I *am* naughty.' A child growing up believing that they are something to the core will have a very different experi-ence to a child that can distance themselves from the act by believing that what they did was wrong but fundamentally they are still an OK person.

Another factor that comes into the mix of our belief systems and how we run our lives is purely physical, and it involves the sex hormones oestrogen and testosterone. Steven Stosny explores this with humour and compassion in his book *How To Improve Your Marriage Without Talking About It*. His research into the psychological effects of these sex hormones shows that oestrogen, the sex hormone that is dominant in women, creates a need for connection with other humans, and it can mean that women's deepest underlying fear is one of abandonment and loss of attachment. In men, whose dominant sex hormone is testosterone, this sets up a drive to achieve and be successful; for most men their deepest fear is that of failure. If we take this back to our existence in caves, these hormones make complete sense, in that for survival it was imperative for women to connect with their mate / children and others in the group, and for men it was important that they did not fail in their task of providing food, shelter and defence. However, in our current society (especially where there are so many people with hormone imbalances), oestrogen can drive people-pleasing and perfectionist behaviours in a bid to increase connection, and testosterone can exacerbate a drive for over-achievement and perfectionism in a bid to protect against possible future failure. These male / female behaviours are obviously not set in stone, there is much crossover as we can see if we stand back and observe society, but they are an important factor to consider when we look at why we behave as we do.

The relatively new science of psycho-endo-neuro-immunology looks at the effect that emotions have on the endocrine (the endocrine system is the system of glands that secrete hormones – our chemical messengers), nervous and immune systems. Research shows that trauma of the mother or father or even from generations further back can be carried down on the DNA, producing physical and emotional effects in the offspring.[93] There is a vital process in the body called methylation, which is what switches genes on and off. This methylation process has an important part to play in reprogramming genes: it can 'wipe' the genes clean for the next generation.[94] It has been observed with profound trauma that the methylation process is damaged and the cell escapes reprogramming, which may create physical changes in the offspring, leading to increased incidences of mental health disorders, cancer and cardiovascular disease etc.[95] [96] [97]

When we are exposed to any form of trauma, and for a small child this can be an experience as seemingly mundane as getting something wrong in class, the stress hormones that it releases into our system, in order to keep us safe, can physically damage our DNA. This DNA is then used in the sperm or the egg to create another life, and the baggage from this defective DNA can have far-reaching physical and emotional consequences down the generations.

Experiences of the foetus in the womb can also have long-term effects. If you have a stressed mother who has high levels of cortisol and adrenalin in her system whilst she is pregnant, this can reset the child's stress response long term. It does not necessarily have to be a major trauma, a low-dose chronic level of stress is enough to reset the physiology of a foetus. Let me explain – if the foetus is exposed to high levels of cortisol whilst it is developing (at this time the foetus is very sensitive and malleable), it can affect gene expression, which in turn affects the development of the HPA (hypothalamus-pituitary-adrenal) axis. The HPA axis will detect that the world is generally not safe due to the mother's stress hormones and so makes the stress response in the foetus over-sensitive in order to keep that little person safe. Babies exposed to stress in utero have been born with a greater risk of attention deficit disorders and depression.[98]

Exposure to chronically high levels of cortisol can change the size of the amygdala and hippocampus in the brain. The amygdala is mostly responsible for processing emotions, so any adverse affects on it can result in a higher percentage of mood disorders.[99]

Interestingly, studies show that massaging babies can reduce cortisol and help to reset their stress response.[100] Professor Judy Atkinson explores this idea in her book *Trauma Trails* and looks at the methods that the indigenous populations in Australia use to process this trauma.

Adverse Child Events, or ACEs, have a powerful impact on the lifestyle, behaviours and physical health of a person throughout life. Associations have been made for increased risk of cancer, heart disease, mental health disorders, increased alcohol and drug use and self-harming. It is interesting to note that in 2007 Bessel van der Kolk, the author of *The Body Keeps the Score*, stated that within a North American context 'people with childhood histories of trauma make up almost our entire criminal justice population.'[101]

BEHAVIOURS THAT A FEARFUL MIND MAY EMPLOY
People-pleasing
This is a survival mechanism – if you upset people you might get thrown out of the tribe. Very relevant when we were living in caves, but still today we have this need for connection in order to make us feel safe. That feeling of *not fitting in* is still equally stressful today and if there is past trauma increasing our fear then the need to fit in is ramped up even more. People-pleasing is a perfect way to disempower ourselves – it sets up within us a constant battle of feeling that you are not OK if you don't say yes and keep everyone happy.

I have a client who has a PhD in people-pleasing: she is a hugely kind and caring person and puts herself at the bottom of the pile and everyone else first all of the time. This mindset also means that she is constantly beating herself up. No matter how positive I am being, she will always manage to turn a question or a statement into a negative about herself. She was totally unaware of this skill (until I pointed it out) and we have spent a long time working on it, increasing her awareness about her mental self-chat. I asked her if she would ever say any of these things to anyone else and she went quite pink and said 'Not in a million years'. So, there is the benchmark: if you wouldn't say it to anyone else, try not to say it to yourself. This takes practice, if you have been used to years of berating yourself. Sometimes people find it helpful to give the negative voice a persona – ideally make it comical (sticky out ears, funny nose, crossed eyes etc) and that way it is easier to dismiss what it is saying when it starts laying into you.

To have good self-esteem we need to have respect for our own beliefs and ideas and truly accept that they are valid; if we are too busy people-pleasing then we are not being genuine to ourselves or others, and there is constant conflict. This can lead to anger and resentment, but in a people-pleaser these emotions can be turned against the self and expressed as depression.

Something that can help the development of our self-esteem is to create a beautiful imaginary pot. I would like you to close your eyes and imagine the colour, the shape, the texture and where it is going to sit inside your body. My pot is a very glossy electric blue and it is perfectly round with a hole in the top, it sits in the centre of my body, just below my rib cage in the inverted V. Take some time to create a fabulous pot, one that makes you smile every time you think of it. Every day I would like you to put something or maybe more than one thing into your pot. Make it something that makes you feel good about yourself, ideally not about achievements, in an ideal world self-esteem should not be about what we have done, although sometimes it is hard to think of things that are not achievement-based. These are some of the things that I have put into my pot:

'I managed to maintain my boundaries with a struggling client and get them to do it themselves rather than leaping in to help.'

'Instead of working all evening I sat down and watched a film with my children.'

'I took the time to rub some cream into my rather dry and uncared for feet.'

'I accepted a compliment by saying thank you rather than protesting and batting it back to the other person.' So often I see people squirming when they receive a compliment and not receiving what essentially you could think of as a gift. Next time someone gives you a compliment, smile and accept this wonderful offering.

Very rarely do I see a client with robust self-esteem who feels OK about themselves. Someone who can comfortably say at all times, '*I am enough*, just as I am ... I don't have to be achieving great things or even little things to be an OK, worthwhile person.'

Where does people-pleasing come from?

Essentially, we are pack animals and we want to fit in; we are also born very dependent upon our parents / caregivers, which means that we are programmed with a survival instinct to please, to ensure that we are not rejected – mother nature's reason for making baby mammals so cute. This survival drive is then compounded by the fact that we are generally praised for being compliant and toeing the line. If you look at it from a more sinister point of view, the underlying subconscious message is: *be good or I won't care for you any more*. As a baby / small child that is pretty life-threatening. Quite understandably, this kind of blanket praise affects our self-esteem as a whole person and can kick the fight / flight in if at any point we are not being 'good'. I am not saying we shouldn't praise children for being good, but the way we say it could be more directed. 'I can see how much effort you put into that picture...' or 'You built that model really carefully...' rather than '*you* are really clever, talented, artistic...' By not linking the praise with the person's core being, we don't manipulate that person's underlying self-esteem. Studies have shown that this kind of praise helps to motivate in a positive way and does not make a child dependent upon praise.

Are you a people-pleaser?
Do you find it hard to say no?

Are you afraid to go out on a limb and voice an opinion that may be contrary to others?

Do you find it easier to just go along with what everyone else wants?

Are you hesitant about taking the initiative?

Do you feel that you can't express your true feelings if there is a risk you might upset someone?

Do you always keep your emotions under control?

Do you go out of your way to keep the peace?

Are you afraid to let people down, even when their demands are unreasonable?

Be aware of the language that you use with yourself: if it contains I should, I ought, I must ... then it is most likely that you are people-pleasing and it is not something that you genuinely want to do. People-pleasing does not make for internal harmony, it usually means that your internal convictions and beliefs are being squashed in order to say and do the 'pleasing' thing.

Harriet Braiker in her book *The Disease to Please* says that the drive to people-please comes from a deep fear of negative emotions – 'fear of rejection, fear of abandonment, fear of conflict or confrontation, fear of criticism, fear of being alone and fear of anger'. Mistakenly, we think that pleasing people will protect us from experiencing any of these uncomfortable emotions. The problem is that unless we have a healthy pot of self-esteem it is very difficult to protect ourselves from feeling rejected, criticised, alone or angry, because our internal voice will do that for us anyway, whatever the outside world is throwing at us.

The next time you are feeling conflicted in a situation and feel that you have to toe the line – be brave, speak up. It does not have to be in a confrontational way; if you are open and honest about the way you are really feeling, people should respect this – and if they don't, remember that is their download that they are working from and not yours. At the end of the day you are doing your best and *that is enough*.

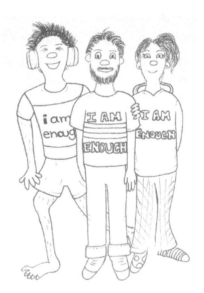

GUILT

When a body is in a state of fear, guilt can become a key player. Guilt keeps the focus continually on the I, which is generally unhelpful. Very often people feel guilty about the small things – something they might have said to someone, or some small thing that they did or didn't do. Often the person feeling so guilty is beating themselves up for absolutely no reason, because the person about whom they are feeling guilt often hasn't even registered that there is a problem. However large your guilt, the only way to process it is to talk to the other person, get it out in the open – all the time it exists as an uncomfortable secret in your heart it is doing damage. If this guilt is a big one and you manage to talk it through with the 'wounded' party and they are not in a place to forgive / reconcile, then you have done your best and it is important to move on. All emotions have an energetic resonance, the negative emotions can cause energetic stagnation in the body, blockage of the chi – chi in traditional Chinese medicine is thought to be the life force of the body and the ultimate measure of its vitality. If chi is blocked it can manifest in physical symptoms, so it is really important to process those negative emotions.

COMMUNICATION IS KEY

In my experience, lack of communication is the root of all misunderstandings, which lead to so much heartache. When we are looking at the world through our own particular lens, it is easy to assume that you know what another person is thinking. The amount of times that this has happened with my husband is laughable; likewise, the other way around, me assuming that he knows what I am thinking and feeling. He has commented to me on various occasions: 'I am not clairvoyant, you need to tell me what you are thinking.' Initially this used to really wind me up because for me it was *so* obvious how I would be feeling about a situation, but that is when I am looking through my lens and nobody else in the entire world has that particular lens. It is important to remember also that we are programmed to focus on the negative as a default, because it means that we are then always prepared for danger and adversity – this is most unhelpful when we are thinking about how others might perceive us.

PERFECTIONISM
Perfectionism – another consequence of the 'I am not enough' download. I am a self-confessed perfectionist, not in all areas of my life, my family will definitely attest to that, but I do have that little voice kicking in on a regular basis if I let it.

What is perfectionism? Here is one definition:

'A person's striving for flawlessness and setting excessively high performance standards, accompanied by overly critical self-evaluations and concerns regarding others' evaluations.'

No wonder so many people are exhausted, driving themselves into the ground in a bid to achieve such high standards. We live in a society where it is impossible not to compare oneself to others. I find it helpful to remember that when we are interacting with people, we are comparing our innermost workings, our doubts, hang-ups, fears and paranoias about ourselves to their outermost exterior, one that has been polished and buffed, censored and perfected. Perfectionism is death to all of our creative potential. It prevents us from going out on a limb, taking a risk, voicing an opinion. I remember being crippled by fear in school at the thought that the teacher might say '… and Kate, what do you think?' My opinions were going to be wrong and stupid. Tie that up with the unforgiving culture of teenagers and you had someone who kept their gaze to the floor in dread that they might be singled out and humiliated. Whilst we remain within the boundaries of worrying what people think, we are totally confined and stuck in our fear.

Brené Brown puts it perfectly: 'Understanding the difference between healthy striving and perfectionism is critical to laying down the shield and picking up your life. Research shows that perfectionism hampers success. In fact, it's often the path to depression, anxiety, addiction, and life paraly-sis.'[102]

So we come back to the message of I am enough, building that confidence so that whatever you are doing is OK; it does not have to be perfect.

THE JOYS OF VICTIMHOOD!

It is important when we start doing this work that we don't start wallowing in 'Woundology', coined by the wonderful Caroline Myss: the 'oh woe is me', victim mentality.

The other day I was really angry about something, stomp-ing across the field with the dogs (getting some space away from other people – safer for them). I noticed that part of me was revelling in that toddler mentality of victimhood *Oh woe is me*, it's not my fault, why can't so and so behave differently – this was a self-righteous disempowering rant, and I suddenly realised that this was fuelling the anger. This was mostly anger at myself for not being able to handle the situation in an adult and exemplary way. If I was going to get my head straight before returning home, a different ap-proach was required.

If we look back at the way that the brain develops when we are tiny, the above mentality is what we develop to help us cope with the world and to keep us safe. Blame everyone else, because if we take responsibility then we may not be so loveable. These stories that we run in our heads become a well-worn neural pathway by the time we are 5, and any stress or threat sees us rushing back to those familiar pat-terns. This was the moment for me to address the down-loads: as much as I felt like stomping and blaming I was going to have to man up and take responsibility.

I think it is important to mention the blame word here – it is very easy to blame our parents / family / circumstances for the challenges that are thrown at us in life, and let them define who we are and how we operate.

We do not, however, have any idea of the downloads from which others are operating and through what sort of lens they are looking at the world.

'Never judge a man till you have walked two moons in his moccasins…'   — Ancient North American tribal saying

A perfect example of this is the other day when I was reminiscing about our childhood with a friend. She was chatting about a particular event that had happened but I remembered it completely differently. Our interpretations of exactly the same event were planets apart – it can be helpful to keep this in mind when there is conflict. At the end of the day it is about taking responsibility for how we choose to react to any event or person. For decades I allowed various events that occurred during my childhood to 'run the show', affecting how I reacted. A lightbulb moment for me was when I attended an event run by Joe Dispenza (if you don't know about Joe Dispenza I highly recommend him); he said, 'Don't give your power away.' I realised that for decades that is exactly what I was allowing to happen and my body was starting to complain.

For the last three years I had suffered with fibromyalgia, a disease where the body produces widespread chronic musculoskeletal pain. Interestingly, in the book *The Secret Language of Your Body* by Inna Segal, this what she writes about fibromyalgia:

Feeling knocked down by life's challenges, overstressed. Lacking in the energy to keep going. Too much to do and not enough time to do it. Life feels like a fight. Feeling stuck and resistant to growth, movement and exploration. Overflowing with sadness, regret, guilt and worry. Feeling depressed, suppressed and on guard.

So many of these applied to me, my body was shouting: in order to heal I needed to break free from my past and stop letting it run the show.

These are the physical symptoms that I can now recognise as my body keeping the score:

Life-long constipation (apologies, probably too much information, but my clients have to share) – inability to let go.

Fibromyalgia – sometimes when I got up in the morning my body felt as if it was 90 it was so stiff and sore.

Sore throats and inability to talk loudly or even shout without developing a sore throat. I was not communicating my needs. In my head I was not entitled to have a voice – be quiet, be a good girl, don't rock the boat and toe the line.

Thyroid issues – all in the throat area.

I was taking exercise, eating a great diet, taking supplements, getting enough good-quality sleep but none of it seemed to make the slightest difference. The problem is, if you have subconscious downloads, which account for 95% of your brain workings, and you are trying to shift a pattern using conscious thought, which accounts for 5% of your brain workings, you can see why you might be on a hiding to nothing. Once I had realised about the 'giving power away' problem, I decided that the only way was to reprogramme those downloads.

Awareness of our downloads is key to enabling us to start re-programming them. When you find yourself overreacting to a relatively benign situation you can bet that it is an old download that is running the show. Sitting quietly and thinking around the problem can often provide insights as to what that past story / experience is; the body has an innate wisdom but so often it gets suppressed because our ego is busy chattering in order to prevent us from digging up painful memories. If you can provide enough stillness and quiet for the mind, insights can often come thick and fast.

For most negative reactions the underlying emotion is fear

– after all, anger / upset is just fear with attitude.

The following are some of the methods that have worked for me.

Emotion code

The book *Emotion Code* by Bradley Nelson was recommended to me by a fellow practitioner, and what a revelation it was. It can be helpful to think of these trapped emotions as balls of energy that are vibrating at an incorrect frequency. When our system cannot process them fully at the time of the event, they can become trapped in the body. It makes sense that by using a magnet you can break up and release these balls of energy and therefore restore physical balance. Many of our trapped emotions have been absorbed from other family members and some of them can be inherited from past generations. Regarding the energy of emotions, you may be interested to look at the work of Dr Masaru Emoto, who demonstrated perfectly how emotional energy can affect physical substances. He performed experiments to show that human emotions, which are vibrations with different frequencies, can affect the molecular structure of water. He exposed different samples of water to different energetic vibrations. Positive emotions such as love, peace, gratitude and truth, or negative emotions such as evil and hate; these emotions were verbalised as well as thought about, so be aware of the power of words. Emoto also exposed the water to harmonious and discordant music. He then froze the different samples of water and photographed the crystal structures. The ones exposed to positive emotions and harmonious music had beautiful regular hexagonal crystals, whereas the ones exposed to negative emotions or discordant music had irregular malformed crystals, which meant that the atoms were not behaving naturally. I will leave you with this thought – our body is approximately 60% water.

Eye movement de-sensitisation and reprocessing (EMDR)
This therapy works on the principle of getting both sides of
the brain to communicate with each other. Similar to REM
(rapid eye movement) sleep, where our eyes move rapidly in
various directions whilst we are sleeping, this links up both
sides of the brain so events can be processed.

When we are talking about an experience, as in therapies
like counselling, we will be engaging the left-hand side of
the brain, the logical and practical side; we are not generally
including the right-hand side of the brain (unless we are
in flashback), where the memory and trauma is stored. For
example, I could say 'It is totally irrational for you to have
your phobia of furry teddies,' and you would say, 'Yes, I
understand that this is a totally irrational fear, but it makes
no difference as to how my body is reacting when I think
about furry teddies.' The problem is that when we are talking about a trauma, we are rarely accessing the memory
of the event that started off the problem in the first place.
Sometimes for trauma, there are flashbacks, where the right
brain is intervening, but because the right side and the left
side are not communicating properly there is no ability to
rationalise the event. Until we can do this it is almost impossible to process the trauma or download and file it properly
in the brain. When processed properly the event will not
produce an inappropriate emotional response, which triggers the fight / flight.

With EMDR, whilst you are accessing the memory (one
of the huge benefits of EMDR is that you don't actually
have to talk about it, you just have to access the memory in
your head), you follow the practitioner's finger / wand with
your eyes (this can also be done auditorily). The movement
is quite fast and it can sometimes be hard work following it
with your eyes, but the release of emotion that it induces is
quite amazing. I can't say that it is an easy or comfortable
process to go through but the results are well worth it.

PSYCH-K®

This is a very effective therapy which also works on the principles of getting both sides of the brain to communicate with each other. This means that you are actually able to communicate directly with the subconscious. The joy of PSYCH-K® is that you can learn how to do this yourself in a three-day workshop so you can help not only yourself but also your family and friends. It has been an invaluable tool in my box. PSYCH-K® works on the principle of muscle testing. Our bodies are energetic beings – energy runs throughout our entire system, if something enters your energetic field which negatively impacts that energy, be it thoughts and emotions or physical substances (including food), it will cause a temporary weakening of the muscles. Once you have established one of your limiting beliefs, in my case one of the big ones was 'I am not safe', you can then reprogramme that belief so it is no longer controlling your reactions to life.

TRE – Trauma Release Exercise

I have found this therapy an extremely helpful adjunct to PSYCH-K® and EMDR as it helps the body to process any trauma held in the tissues. Trauma Release Exercise (TRE) is a technique developed by David Berceli. This technique again enables us to process locked-in emotional trauma. Put simply, when we are in fight / flight mode the stress hormones create a certain amount of muscle tension; if these unconscious patterns of muscle tension are not released then it can lead to long-term muscular and structural problems in the body. If you observe animals that are stressed / excited, they often start to shake; our spaniels are a perfect example of this – when they sense it is time for a walk, adrenalin courses through their systems and they shake, this helps to release muscle tension and also to burn off the adrenalin. TRE is a set of exercises that stress the muscles temporarily and then allows a natural reflex of vibration and shaking. This is a really easy process to learn and the joy of it is that you do not have to be thinking about any of your stresses for it to work – the body will process it for you.

Biodynamic Craniosacral Therapy
This is another effective therapy that has helped to keep me going. This is a very gentle therapy (the first time I had it I really wondered what was going on as the therapist did not seem to be doing anything but I can assure you the results were hugely beneficial). This therapy tunes into the central nervous system and can detect any emotional or physical blockages that exist, which it then releases.

Bio-Resonance
A therapy that is based upon the principle that unhealthy cells or organs will emit a different electromagnetic wavelength from their healthy counterparts. By detecting these altered wavelengths, bio-resonance can be used to accurately diagnose disease in the body. These wavelengths can then be changed back to their normal frequency, restoring balance.

EFT
This therapy arose from the idea that 'The cause of all negative emotions is a disruption in the body's energy system.' Whilst tapping on acupressure meridian points, we can help to release the disruptions and blockages by speaking out loud a statement of what the problem / feeling is and then following it with a statement that shows complete acceptance and acknowledgement of the issue. For example, 'Even though I am terrified about giving this presentation, I deeply love and accept myself.' For some, the last bit of the statement is too difficult to say so it can be adjusted to 'I acknowledge and accept these feelings.' This therapy is very easy to learn and is particularly good to do with children.

Writing to connect with your inner child

If you are a fan of writing the following process can also be very helpful, and again it works on linking up both sides of the brain. We can have a chat with our subconscious by writing with both our right and left hands. I had quite a few conversations with my own 'inner child'. Talking as me, I wrote with my right hand (I am right-handed), and then when I was listening for the opinions of my inner child, I wrote them with my left hand. This process is explained brilliantly in the book *Recovery of Your Inner Child* by Lucia Capacchione. I started to have chats with the little Kate – she was quite feisty and rather pissed off with the fact that I had been toeing the line so much and that my life was all rather serious and quite frankly from her point of view very dull. She wanted a bit more craziness and fun. This is a work in progress, much helped by my lovely tribe of friends.

Writing can be employed in many helpful ways when trying to work out what is really going on; these lightbulb moments can be an important part of the healing process. Writing for some does not come naturally, but just keep at it, even if you start off with a shopping list, and just put down anything that is going on in your head.

Another way of employing writing is, when we are angry or upset with someone, we can write them a letter in which we let it all pour out. This can be a way of really getting down to the nitty-gritty of the problem – I don't suggest that we actually send the letter, but a ceremonial burning of it to release all those emotions can be very therapeutic. Another use for letters is if we need to voice an opinion or address an issue with someone, something that we find hard to talk about, and in the heat of the moment it might come out wrong, or in my case we are sobbing so hard we can't get the words out. Writing it down can mean that we say exactly what we are meaning in a calm and accurate way, without getting hijacked by emotions.

THE SIGNIFICANCE OF CONNECTION

It's all about energy

This is where we get into the proper woo-woo stuff, I used to think it was all woo-woo until I started looking into quantum physics, not that I can get my head around much of it, but all of these amazing phenomena are scientifically proven.

In the words of Albert Einstein: 'Everything is energy and that is all there is to it. Match the frequency of the reality you want and you cannot help but get that reality. It can be no other way. This is not philosophy. This is physics.'

An extremely important element to emotional wellbeing is being aware of our connectedness. We have developed a modern society where human connection is not given the priority it should be, and we are all too busy being individual warriors putting on a good face and suppressing emotion. There are many forms of connection which I will explore below.

Loss of connection, whether it be energetically, emotionally or physically, is stressful for the body.

Loss of connection with self

What are your core values? It can be really helpful to think about your own core values and make sure that they don't get hijacked by society's expectations or individual people's views.

To discover what your core values are, it can be useful to remember a time when you were happy and fulfilled, and work out which core values were being satisfied. You can also do this in reverse: think of a time that sticks out when you were angry, upset etc … which of your core values were being violated?

Once you have established your core values try to ensure that your day includes activities that feed them.

What is your Ikigai?
This is the Japanese word for 'reason for being' or raison d'etre. It is well known that when people retire, they are more likely to develop some kind of chronic complaint or have a heart attack. Work provides mental and social stimulation and unless our retirement is full of a sense of purpose, a reason to get out of bed in the morning and ongoing social interaction, this can have a profound effect on our body's ability to maintain a healthy balance. Ikigai does not have to be a grand plan, for some it may be the ability to play with the grandchildren, weed that flower bed, help a friend out or cook a really delicious meal. Whatever it is, it needs to give you a sense of purpose and fulfilment.

Playing the 'I'll be happy when...' *game*
Fulfillment doesn't always live on the other side of a person, place, thing or accomplishment.
- I'll be happy when I have got a bit more money
- I'll be happy when we move house
- I'll be happy when I have lost that weight
- I'll be happy when I have got that assignment done
- I'll be happy when it is the weekend

It is very easy to play the 'I'll be happy when...' game, but the journey is just as important. Some of these 'whens' may never happen, but thinking this way can mean that we wish away our lives. Although you might be in a really tough situation at this precise moment, it is helpful to endeavour to enjoy the journey rather than focus on the point at which that situation might be changed.

Is this life serving me?
Here are some questions that might be helpful to ask:
Do you feel in control of your life most of the time?
Are you mentally and / or physically being stretched in

ways that give you a sense that life is meaningful?

Are you achieving things and feeling competent in at least one major area of your life?

Do you have a reason (about which you care deeply) to get out of bed in the morning?

Do you have an intimate relationship in your life – one where you can be totally physically and emotionally accepted for who you are by at least one other person?

Do you feel emotionally connected to others?

Do you feel connected to some part of the outside community?

If you have a few NOs in there, it might be beneficial to take action.

In the book *Blue Zones* by Dan Buettner, he discovered, by studying areas around the world where people tend to live much longer than average, that one of the key ingredients to longevity was having a sense of connection to other people, not just close family but to the wider community. Feeling that you belong to a group of people who have the same values as you makes it much easier to stick to those values and be comfortable with who you are.

Loneliness statistics from Age UK – 2014
Over 1 million older people say they are always lonely or often feel lonely.

Loneliness increases the likelihood of mortality by 26%.

Nearly half of older people (49% of the 65+s) say that television or pets are their main form of company.

It is estimated that by 2025 the amount of lonely over-50s is set to reach 2 million in the UK.

Loneliness for our health can be as harmful as smoking 15 cigarettes a day: it promotes the progression of heart disease and high blood pressure.

People with a high degree of loneliness are twice as likely to develop Alzheimer's.

Lonely people have a higher risk of depression and suicide.

We are tribal animals at the end of the day and if we feel alone it will switch on our fight / flight mechanisms. This would explain why loneliness is so bad for our health.

The way that we interact with each other has changed beyond recognition, even from when I was a child – this poem really struck a chord with me.

Call On Me

we don't call on each other anymore
we all live too far away
and now impromptu visits worry you
might interrupt my day
you do not wake me up
on weekends
with screams pitched
to my bedroom glass
do not ring my doorbell
more than once
politer now
step off the mat
now we must plan to meet
in diaries
don't dance in pjs /
share the bed
you do not comb my hair
for hours, to practise plaits
- drink tea instead
I love you still, my friends
I count our meetings down like holidays

but dream each time the doorbell rings
it's you, just called to play

— Hollie McNish

The irony with technology is that it is ever easier to stay connected but this does not substitute for actual physical connection: having someone in the same room is so much more beneficial, and there is so much more to interaction than just the words.

Energy field of your heart
The electromagnetic field that is emitted by our heart is 60 times stronger than that which is emitted from our brain. Due to the incredible work done by the HeartMath Institute we know that there is more information going from the heart to the brain than the brain to the heart. The heart is instrumental in surveillance of our surroundings, due to the fact that its electromagnetic field extends approximately five feet out from the body. Experiments show that if you are standing close to someone and your hearts' electromagnetic fields cross over and there is coherence between the two bodies, the heart rates will start to beat at the same time. When I first discovered this, I was rather skeptical but also blown away with this idea. How incredible that we can affect something so fundamental as the heart rate of somebody else by just standing close to them. I tried it with my husband and children and it really does work. This exchange of energy is thought to be a major part of the healing process in practices such as reiki, qigong, contact and distance healing.

This electromagnetic field can be affected by emotions, the energy of compassion and love can be transmitted from one individual's body to another, as can the emotions of anger and fear – so take care who you spend time with.

Beware the energy vamp
It is easy for other people to interfere with our energy field. When you spend time with someone and you come away feeling totally drained, not necessarily through what they have said, it is probably because you are being energetically zapped – that person is meddling with your energy field. I can assure you that most of the time this will be done completely unconsciously by the other person. If you know that you are going to have to spend time with an energy zapper, you can mentally put a protective bubble around yourself – make it whatever colour you like and made of whatever material works. For a more in-depth look at this type of protection I urge you to look at the work of Adrian Incledon-Webber. Alternatively, many people find it helpful to wear crystals on their person to help with grounding (see page 223) and protection.

Perils and blessings of technology
It is fabulous that we can now contact anyone in the world at the drop of a hat, and that we have access to knowledge and information with a few taps on a keyboard. However, 90% of all the data in the world has been generated in the last two years and the human brain is being bombarded. Look around when you are walking along the street: how many people are looking at their phones reading texts, replying to emails or talking to people far distant. Apart from the damage that it does to our necks, putting a huge amount of extra strain on the muscles, it seems that we are now not allowed any downtime – every minute of the day has to be filled.

Not being attached to a phone gives you more space to connect with your surroundings and be in the moment, it seems to slow down time. The irony of this constant busyness and multitasking is that our overall productivity is reduced. Life has speeded up to a point where most of us have overload, which leads to excess amounts of cortisol; this adversely affects brain function, particularly memory, and keeps us on the hamster wheel of fight / flight, where there is less time to reach out and connect with others.

The power of words
Everything around us has a resonant frequency and this includes words: the more positive the language we use the higher the frequency, which raises our vibration. This directly affects our cells, it sounds woo-woo but it is just physics. If you look up 'Cymatics: Chladni plate' with Nigel Stanford on YouTube you can see a beautiful visual of this.

Clients often say to me 'I *am* so stupid … or exhausted or sad or anxious etc' – when we speak this way it is incredibly disempowering, it is like we embody that negativity and have no choice in the matter. Distancing ourselves from the event / thing means that you retain the power to change it.

I did such a stupid thing

I really need a rest

I choose to feel sad at the moment

I am excited at the moment – in the body there is very little difference between excitement and anxiety, all the same hormones will be running, so by continuing to tell yourself that your anxiety is excitement this can help to change the mindset.

Unnecessary apologising is another problematic semantic trap that many of us fall into (especially the British); saying sorry for situations that we are just not responsible for makes us feel like a victim, and it gives other people the impression that we lack confidence, so they are much less likely to respect our boundaries.

The science of smiling
Going back to the fact that our mind and body are

inextricably linked, it has been discovered that smiling creates a happiness feedback loop. Exercising our zygomaticus major muscle and orbicularis oculi muscle (smiling muscles for you and I) actually makes us feel happier. This is how it works: when something good happens, our brain is happy which produces endorphins (feel-good hormones) and this sends a message to our face muscles so that we smile. When our smile muscles contract, they send a message back to the brain, which stimulates our reward system and makes us feel even happier. So, we can miss out the first part if we are struggling to get the happy event and just skip to the smile (even if you don't feel like it). Try it, I promise it makes you feel better, not just a Mona Lisa glimmer – go for the full-on cheesy grin.

This is even more effective if you do it in front of the mirror because we all have mirror neurons. Mirror neurons are a very important mechanism for what makes humans sociable. If you google images of human smiling faces, you will find yourself automatically smiling. Mirror neurons are activated when we perform an action, but they are also activated when we observe an action, so it is a really good idea to hang out with smiley people. I experimented on the tube one day to see how many people I could get to smile – the biggest problem is getting anyone to catch your eye (and not being arrested for suspect behaviour). Everyone is very busy being physically disconnected (in protection mode), even though they might be technologically connected. However, with the people I did manage to engage, it really did work – smiling is infectious.

'Sometimes your joy is the source of your smile, but sometimes your smile can be the source of your joy.'
— Thich Nhat Hanh

The hormone of connection
It has been scientifically proven that kindness improves our health and this is mostly attributable to the hormone oxytocin, otherwise named the 'love' or 'cuddle' hormone. Oxytocin is produced in buckets during childbirth and having sex, vital as it is for mother–child bonding and fidelity. Men and women treated with oxytocin are far less likely to 'stray' than those with lower levels.

Witnessing acts of kindness triggers our body to produce oxytocin, which also helps to relax us by lowering stress hormones, heart rate and blood pressure.[103] The more oxytocin there is around the longer you will live.

Oxytocin can help with depression, because it causes an increase of endorphins in the body.[104]

Oxytocin can reduce pain – conservative estimates show that approximately 15% of the population in the UK experience chronic pain, taking a huge toll on human experience, let alone productivity. It is not known if the pain-relieving action is due to oxytocin's positive effect on mood and anxiety, but it gives no side effects like other pain-relieving medications. You would have thought that generating oxytocin in the body would be being pursued as an effective pain relief solution but you can't patent something that naturally occurs in the body and this approach does not involve giving pills so is unlikely to catch on with medicine at the moment.

According to research from Emory University, when you are kind to another person your brain's pleasure and reward centres light up, due to the production of oxytocin. It is as if you were the recipient of the good deed – not the giver. This phenomenon is called the 'helper's high'.

Best ways to increase oxytocin
Hugging – wherever I can I will always hug because it does both of us good even if the other person thinks me a little forward. This also goes for hugging and physical contact

with animals too. With Covid-19 raging, hugging is out which I find particularly difficult; I am hoping that one of the silver linings of this very challenging situation is that a greater sense of community and togetherness will rise out of this unprecedented crisis.

Other benefits of hugging show:

It increases dopamine (motivation and reward brain chemical) and serotonin (happy hormone).

It reduces stress by making us feel safe, this means lower cortisol levels, which in turn can lower blood pressure, blood sugar levels and muscle tension.

Less stress means a more effective immune system.

It releases endorphins, these not only make you feel good but also help to reduce pain.

Make eye contact with people – something easy to forget when we are all glued to our screens.

If you meditate, focus on others – there are some great loving kindness meditations online.

Join a club / class – be involved with other people.

Touch – have a massage or give one, or even just hold someone's hand. Skin is the major interface between our body and the outside world, containing a network of nerve cells that detects and relays information about our changing environment. When the touch is pleasurable, the feedback to the body is positive and calming. Touch has been found to have huge health benefits, from the physical and emotional development of babies and children,[105] the reduction of pain and stress,[106] the boosting of the immune system[107] and the decrease in negative behavioural symptoms observed in patients with dementia.[108] It has also been shown that touch is an accurate way to communicate emotions.[109] Hertenstein found that emotions such as anger, disgust, love, gratitude, sympathy, happiness and sadness could all be communicated to a blindfold participant with an accuracy of 78%.

More Sex Please – sex is something that is hugely beneficial from a physical and psychological stance, but it can also be a complicated matter. If you are struggling in this area, I urge you to read Esther Perel's books – *Mating in Captivity* and *State of Affairs*. She discusses this topic with huge compassion and wisdom.

Release your emotions – better out than in is always my motto, and suppression of emotions has been found to suppress oxytocin. Watching a weepy / feel-good film can be very beneficial, or booking in for a boxing session if there are pent-up emotions. Depression can be anger that is turned against oneself – it often happens to those gentle, sensitive individuals who feel that it is not acceptable to express it.

Join a group in the community, be it a sport, choir, painting, writing etc, anything that promotes that sense of teamwork or being in a group; we are after all a herd animal.

Surround yourself with the right kind of people – I am blessed to have some incredibly supportive family and friends, people that I can be totally vulnerable with and who I know will not judge me. There are times when we just need that extra bit of support, and the following occasion is one where my brother came to the rescue. I was having to give a presentation in London to a high-powered group of people, over which I had been sweating for a few days – not good for the adrenals. I asked my brother to send me calm vibes and this is what I received.

'I hope that by tomorrow you won't need any calming vibes, but I will send off a small party of them to sashay the mile or so from Clerkenwell south to Fleet Street – some of them wear green velvet slippers – so you will be able to recognise them. They will be given instructions to waft in through the window and form a comfortable cushion on which you can lean – a bit like a pack of well-behaved and adoring Labradors.'

The right tribe

Over time I have gathered around me the most incredible tribe of wonderful, wise, intuitive, loyal and empathic women. You know the ones where you can talk about your deepest, most uncomfortable secrets and you know that they won't judge, or turn away or play the game of one-upmanship. They have helped me enormously, not least because they question my beliefs when I am bogged down by the smudged lenses through which I am observing the world.

As part of my work as a Nutritional Therapist, I give workshops that look at nutrition but also lifestyle, and of course stress – these workshops take a good part of the day and usually by the time I have finished I am fairly drained. As I drive home from the workshop my 'vulnerability hangover' usually appears. I can't take credit for this spectacular phrase, it came from the wonderful Brené Brown. If you don't have her in your life, I strongly recommend her – start with her TED talk on having the courage to show your vulnerabilities.

So, there I was driving along with my 'vulnerability hangover' – it went something like this:

'There were a couple of people who were rather quiet during the workshop...

I am sure that they were bored?

Was I too scientific or was I too woo-woo?

Did I shock them when I started talking about sex?

Perhaps they didn't like the lunch?

I didn't get good vibes from that person, did I say something to upset her?'

And on it goes...

I was talking about my vulnerability hangover with a very wise friend and she astutely pointed out that even if everyone who had attended the workshop had written a 3-page email extolling the virtues of the day, there would always be that little voice piping up with a '… but …'

This was a bit of a revelation: no matter how well I had done that little voice was always going to attempt to undermine me. I am now very mindful of this self-sabotaging mechanism that might try to eat away at my self-esteem. Whenever it even thinks about piping up I am usually right down on it like a ton of bricks – most of the time I manage this and sometimes can even laugh at some of the outrageous things that it tries to throw at me.

Having the right people to give you love and support is incredibly valuable, they are the ones who are more comfortable in their skins, not comparing or competitive, and above all they have time to listen.

Connection to faith
In addition to physically connecting with people, it can be really helpful to develop some sort of spirituality. I don't have a formal religion but I do believe that there is a huge supply of assistance that is available to us all, if we can trust and ask for it. Studies have shown that there are benefits to health for those who attend a religious service, even if it is just once a month. As I haven't quite worked out where I stand with organised religion, I have a couple of different groups I go to in order to connect. One is a group of girls that I meet with, to talk about life and stuff, we usually have some homework – reading a useful book (for example *Biology of Belief* by Bruce Lipton) which we discuss. This group is affectionately known by my family as the Witches Coven. It is a group of girls who have all been through various trials and life lessons – their courage and wisdom is outstanding and I feel very blessed to be included. The other group is one set up after having taken part in one of Lynne McTaggart's Power of Eight seminars. A group of like-minded girls meet and send specific healing intention to anyone, either

someone who is in the room or who we know of that is in need of help (we always have their permission). I always come away from these sessions buzzing with energy and excitement. Lynne's experiments show that it is not only the people who are receiving the intention that benefit, those that send it also benefit and I can without doubt testify to this.

Connection with our body

It is very easy with the busyness of 21st-century living to stop listening to our bodies and just be in our heads the whole time. At this point I feel that it may be useful to mention the work of Candace Pert, who wrote *Molecules of Emotion*. She discovered that every cell in our body contains receptors for our brain chemicals, the very same brain chemicals that are produced to create an emotion. So, the body and the mind are inextricably linked: if you are feeling sad all of your cells 'feel' sad, if you are happy all of your cells 'feel' happy. Dr Pert helps us to understand the mechanism by which stress or any negative emotion can cause our bodies to produce all sorts of symptoms. If we can view these symptoms as communication that all is not well, and we are prepared to listen, then we are well on the path to healing. Dr Pert went even further by teaching that the effect of the mind went beyond the body via consciousness. This explains how individuals and groups can affect each other physically and emotionally. Sadly, at the time her hypotheses were met with derision by the conventional medical world; things are slowly changing but we are generally still stuck in the place of a pill for an ill.

Some ways to help connect with our body are:

Walk barefoot whenever you can

Moisturise your body – really appreciate what a great job it is doing for you

Meditate

Be aware of your breathing

Get into the habit of asking your body what it needs and really give yourself some space to listen

Check in with what your fight / flight response is doing – perhaps have a scale to keep track

Practise yoga / tai chi / qigong / pilates

Your posture communicates more than you think
When we watch animals in nature, we see an amazing display of emotion – they are happy to wear their hearts on their sleeves. Animals that are in a threat situation will often try to make themselves look as big as possible, their fight / flight might be running high but in a bid for survival they need to look threatening. In humans if we are feeling fearful, the power postures can be really helpful – hands on hips making us bigger or hands behind the back exposing our internal organs, displaying to the world that we feel secure enough to do that. When we are feeling insecure and unsure, we can do the opposite, arms across the body, legs crossed, we fold into ourselves, and become as small as possible, almost like we are not worthy to be occupying space. This has an impact on how we are perceived by others: we give off 'weak' cues so others feel that they can dominate us. What is even more interesting is that these body postures also have an impact upon our thoughts and feelings by affecting hormone levels. It is no surprise that when we are exhibiting insecure body postures our cortisol levels will rise and when we exhibit the more powerful postures our cortisol levels lower. There is nothing more stressful than feeling disempowered, and if you stand or sit in a disempowered way, this reinforces the message to your body that this is the case. This is a situation where 'fake it till you make it' comes in. Even if we are feeling unsure or insecure, it can help to make ourselves bigger, keep our arms away from the body or behind our back, don't cross our legs, take up space in the world: we deserve to be there.

I practise this when I have a scary presentation to make and it really does help, although be aware of how other people are reacting to your 'power postures', as it can be intimidating for them and that may not be your intention.

Fear-based behaviour is something that is inbuilt to keep us safe, but I find the words of Susan Jeffers most helpful:

'We cannot escape fear. We can only transform it into a companion that accompanies us on all our exciting adventures… Take a risk a day – one small or bold stroke that will make you feel great once you have done it.'[110]

The importance of movement

'And we should consider every day lost on which we have not danced at least once.' — Nietzsche

We have been given these incredible machines that are purpose-built for movement in hugely impressive ways. The problem is that many of us are not taking advantage of these incredible machines. The fault lies mainly with all the labour-saving devices that we have invented to make life easier. It is now so easy to be sedentary, especially when we are feeling exhausted. In Dan Buettner's book *Blue Zones*, he found that in many of the communities where people were living well beyond the average lifespan, they are not using remote controls, leaf blowers, hoovers and kitchen gadgets, cars etc. Their lives naturally contain more movement, and if they do partake in intentional exercise it is something that they enjoy. If you are not a natural mover finding an exercise that floats your boat can be a challenge; it can be intimidating to join a class although I highly recommend it, as it helps to create connection. If you are not a people person and like your own company, a vigorous bop around the kitchen can be just as good – find that piece of music that you just can't not move to.

There are also increased benefits of exercising out in nature: research has found that people are more likely to exercise for longer, and if they are running or walking, the terrain will be more varied, which uses a wider variety of muscles (very hard to go downhill on a treadmill). There is a 50% increased benefit to people's mental health if you are out in nature and it is a lot cheaper than going to a gym.

The effect of dance on the body
As well as dance being good for balance and coordination, muscle-tone and the cardiovascular system, dancing is also hugely beneficial for the brain. The cerebellum, involved in balance, equilibrium, muscle-tone, and the coordination of voluntary motor movement, can easily get underused. As they say, 'Use it or lose it' when it comes to brain function. As we get older, balance is one of the things that we can lose first, leading to all sorts of falls and breakages. Dancing will help to develop muscle memory and also brain memory if you are trying to remember a routine. I am part of a group that does street dance every week and it is a huge challenge for me to remember the routine. Just in case you had visions of me spinning on my head, I want to allay any illusion that I can perform anything remotely cool or impressive.

The effect of music on the body
In *The Mozart Effect* Don Campbell explores the idea of the healing effect of music upon the body and mind.
'Music helps plants grow, drives our neighbours to distraction, lulls children to sleep, and marches men to war…'
Music can:
- Affect our heart rate and reduce blood pressure[111]
- Slow our brain waves[112]
- Reduce stress hormones[113]
- Boost our immune system[114]

- Reduce depression[115]

There are many pieces of music that make me want to move and I often have a jig about at my standing-up desk whilst sending emails. If I want a piece of music that gives me goosebumps it is the 'Prisoners' Chorus' from *Fidelio* by Beethoven.

Singing can also provide the above benefits, especially if it is done within a group. It boosts serotonin, oxytocin and endorphins. Endorphins are our natural opiates, which act as pain relievers and mood enhancers without the side effects. Singing has also been found to have a balancing effect by stimulating the right temporal lobe, the side of the brain responsible for intuition and creativity, something that can take rather a back seat with the huge amount of information that has to be processed in the left-hand side.

Connection with nature

I hear many clients say: 'But I have tried *everything…*' – my answer would be: 'But have you tried nature?' mother earth provides a very powerful healing energy if we can connect with her again. Almost all elements of nature have healing properties within, from the soil to the rocks to the plants to the atmosphere. Our body is connected to mother earth, our heart rhythms and brain waves naturally resonate at the same frequency as the earth's magnetic resonance. Events that happen on the sun's surface can affect us physically, and research has shown that there are significant correlations between hospital admissions and solar geomagnetic activity. It is also well known that A&E departments will increase their staff during full moons. Sadly, we are more and more cut off from nature: we live in hermetically sealed houses, children don't play outside so much, as the lure of a screen is far more seductive. We drive around in cars, many of us exercise in gyms and we wear footwear that cuts us off from the charge of the earth.

The importance of grounding / earthing

This is the process of actually allowing your skin to be in physical contact with mother earth, something that has happened for tens of thousands of years, when the human body walked, stood, sat and slept in contact with the ground. Relatively recently in the history of evolution we have all become disconnected, walking in rubber / plastic-soled shoes, sleeping in raised insulated beds and living in electrically insulated houses.

In the food chapter I talk about antioxidants and how important they are for dampening down free radical damage in the body. Antioxidants are effectively a supply of free electrons that can be donated to the wayward free radicals to stop them from trying to steal electrons from other atoms and causing damage.

Mother earth has an unending supply of free electrons to offer, a supply that is being constantly replenished by natural phenomena like lightning strikes and solar radiation. If we have direct skin contact with the earth we benefit from this supply of electrons, which can be transferred from the earth through the skin and into the body. Any which way we can find to get into contact with the earth will be beneficial: at every opportunity take your shoes off outside, especially when you are at the beach – swimming in the sea is probably one of the most grounding activities you can indulge in. Water is particularly good for conducting those free electrons.

Interestingly many of the eastern traditions of body maintenance, like qigong, tai chi and yoga, are practised with bare feet, and there is an emphasis on visualising roots growing from your feet down into the ground. Earthing has been proven to help a huge number of ailments. As discussed before, inflammation, a process that happens in all disease, produces high levels of free radical damage, so being earthed can help to dampen the inflammatory process. Earthing has also been found to help rebalance cortisol levels. A study in

2004 observed the results of subjects with sleep issues, pain, anxiety and depression when they slept on a grounding mat (this can now be purchased as a sheet to put on the bed). The results showed that there was natural realignment of the circadian rhythm, which improved all of the above health issues. Additionally, sleeping grounded can increase melatonin levels by an average of 8%.

Creating also grounds us, and we do not have to be a fabulous artist to create. Creating could be anything from colouring in, sewing, cooking, gardening, singing, writing, doodling, humming, playing an instrument, dancing round the kitchen ... the list is endless. Anything that brings you joy and lifts your soul. *The Artist's Way* by Julia Cameron is a really helpful book; she recommends journalling at the beginning of each day to start the creative flow. If you are not a writer, journalling can sound challenging but stick with it, just write anything that comes into your head no matter how crazy or trivial. One thing that I will say is that we need brain space for creativity: constant sensory overload kills creativity. See RESOURCES for items to help grounding.

Energy of trees
Trees like all living things have an energy field, and they can communicate with each other. If you are interested please look at the Interconnectivity Tree Research Project. Not only do trees provide the earth with oxygen and clean our air but they also can elicit positive emotions in humans. That is why tree hugging is such a good idea.

Energetics of food
This idea follows through to foods, which generally have a water content. The meat of an animal that has had a happy relaxed life is going to have a far better structure / energy than that of an animal that has been maltreated. Likewise the growing conditions of fruits and vegetables can also

impact their energetics: has it been allowed to grow at its own pace or has it been squashed in with other plants, which stresses it, rendering it more likely to produce plant toxins? Has its growth been affected with growth promoters or growth inhibitors, has it had chemical pesticides / herbicides sprayed on it, or been picked / harvested thousands of miles away and artificially ripened on its journey? The case is made for locally produced ethically raised food. The Slow Food Movement set up in the 1980s by Carlo Petrini hoped to reignite people's interest in food, and raise awareness about how our food choices affect our health and the health of the planet.

I guess what I am saying is that there is so much going on in the universe on an energetic level that profoundly affects our bodies. I hope that the above has given you some insight into the extra-curricular activity that is going on around us all of the time.

'Watch with glittering eyes the whole world around you because the greatest secrets are always hidden in the most unlikely places. Those who don't believe in magic will never find it.'

— Roald Dahl

12

'LET FOOD BE THY MEDICINE'

– HIPPOCRATES

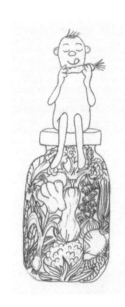

We are hardwired to gorge as a survival mechanism, so don't be too hard on yourself when the wheels fall off. During our hunter-gatherer times, the only sugar that we might have bumped into would be ripe fruit or, if you were very fortunate and had the skill to extract the honey, a bee nest.

To our bodies, sugar equals energy and energy equals survival. This as a starting point in our current environment is hugely unhelpful.

WHY ARE WE EATING?

There is a huge difference between physical hunger and hedonic hunger, the hunger that is trying to plug an emotional hole. I am guilty as charged: I still eat for reasons other than being hungry – usually for me it is sadness or tiredness. I have come a long way from wolfing down a pile of chocolate biscuit cake or consuming a whole Mr Kipling treacle tart at the age of 8. My mother's enquiry as to the whereabouts of the said treacle tart led to a 'Beam me up Scottie' moment – head hanging in shame.

Ever since I can remember I have had issues with food. As a child I was not fat, I would say 'squidgy' would fit the bill. I remember sitting in the bath hunched over at the age of about 7 with little rolls on my stomach, and being told 'That looks disgusting,' and I remember feeling such shame: how could I possibly be OK if I looked disgusting? At 11 I went off to boarding school (now that is a hotbed for creating eating disorders) with all sorts of shapes and sizes, but in my eyes, the cool pretty ones were always skinny. I was no longer squidgy, looking back at photos, but I thought that I was. This ingrained message in my head was compounded by messages from the environment: where were the squidgy girls in the magazines? Thank god we didn't have social media then.

I longed to be thin but just couldn't keep away from the biscuits and cakes, and I now recognise that the more I work on releasing my emotional baggage the less fixation I have with food. At the age of 12, I was given a steroid injection for problems with my knees. Steroids can have a profound effect upon our gut bacteria and very often lead to problems with yeast. Thus started my 20-year dance with a yeast overgrowth, which needed feeding. Yeast loves sugar and I became a sugar junky, but it wasn't just sugar: I craved the worst of both worlds, a combination of sugar and fat. I was a chocolate girl, and we are not talking the 85% stuff.

At the age of 30 I went to see a Nutritional Therapist; having had 3 babies in quick succession my body was feeling exhausted. This was the beginning of an incredible journey – I was gripped by what the Nutritional Therapist told me, ordered Patrick Holford's *Optimum Nutrition Bible*, read it from cover to cover and had the lightbulb moment of 'This is what I want to do.' I signed up to train as a Nutritional Therapist, having first got my Chemistry A Level at a local girls' school – don't do this if you don't want to feel really old! Three years of weekends up and down to London while my children were small – huge and never-ending gratitude to my uncomplaining husband who was supportive and encouraging. Every lecture was a revelation about the miraculousness of our bodies and I started to really understand what was going on in my own.

Food will always be a comfort to me when things get overwhelming, but I am now aware of it. I have also made peace with my body and make a point of acknowledging its amazingness on a daily basis. When I look at my tummy which has stretch marks and is wobbly I have to remember that it has helped to create three amazing human beings and I wouldn't swap that for the world. If I start to put on weight now, I know it is because I am stressed, my body has gone into protection mode and is hanging on to those calories for dear life. I have also discovered with some of my weight-loss clients that if they are the sort of people who have always been a good girl / boy, toeing the line, absorbing everyone else's angst and trauma, their body will hang on to the weight as protection from the outside world. Until these people start having a voice, begin looking after themselves and stop being a magnet for all those who need to off-load, their body will stay in protection mode and so will the weight.

On a more practical level here are some things that have helped me.

In the past, one of the most challenging types of meals that fell into my danger zone were those times when there were lots of delicious dishes spread over the table in front of me and everyone helped themselves. I would set off with good intentions and give myself a sensible portion and start chomping through it. I would then have an empty plate in front of me (having been taught to always finish what is on my plate, this has set up a powerful download about not wasting food) with lots of tempting goodies still left in the middle of the table that are all shouting at me 'Just a little bit more, I'm sure you are not really full.' Now if you are a consummate finisher-upper (mustn't waste food), half-finished plates are a real source of stress. I often ate things rather than throw them away, even though I wasn't hungry and sometimes didn't even particularly like what I was finishing up. In a bid to make it easier for ourselves and if at all possible, put all the dishes out on the side, help yourself and then bring it to the table so at least when you have finished you don't have food right in front of you as a temptation.

Another issue that I find makes it harder for me to stay on track, and seemingly for many clients too, is what we have in our cupboards. If we buy the things that we are trying to avoid and they are sitting in the cupboard they will shout at us – 'Just one won't hurt you know you want to.' If I am tired / emotional my resolve starts to crumble, and before I know it I am heading for the cupboard in a zombie-like state. Of course, just *one* doesn't fit the bill because as soon as that sugar kicks in I become like a drug addict and need more until the packet is finished. The adage 'everything in moderation' is not helpful when it comes to sugar; even a little can trigger all those cravings. Many clients I talk to say: 'Well I need to have it in the house for the children.' This is a tricky one as we all want to be popular care givers and feeding our children the food that they want is one of the ways to achieve this. Unfortunately for my children their Mum was a bit of a food obsessive so excuses like 'Oh the shop had run out' or 'I forgot' were alibis. I could get away with this when they were little but now they are older and wiser they generally go along with it. I am not sure if this exemplary behaviour extends to when they are at university but they are old enough to make their own choices. I found it was a chipping-away process: I didn't suddenly stop stocking everything high-sugar and processed overnight, but in time things that we used to have in the house just didn't feature any more.

FOOD DIARY – CAN BE A VERY USEFUL TOOL

When clients come to see me, they fill in a three-day diary and once we get past the 'I am so embarrassed about what I am eating' thing it can be a real eye-opener. I applaud clients for their honesty (it also makes my job a lot easier) and I hope that from reading this book so far you will see I am in absolutely no position to be judging.

When people are faced with, in writing, what they are consuming, it can be most enlightening, they often say 'I had no idea I was eating so many slices of bread or drinking so many cups of coffee / tea or so little water...'

When it comes to a healthy diet it is unhelpful to think that a one-size-fits-all approach works. If we look at the different genetic makeups, the huge diversity of gut bacteria and the widely differing environments that we live in, it would be naive for me to recommend one specific way of eating and expect it to work for everyone. However, in my humble opinion and experience, I think that removing / reducing grains, legumes and sugar, increasing vegetables and ensuring good-quality protein consumption (this does not mean large amounts of meat) works for a great number of people. The question of whether you reduce or remove the grains and legumes slightly depends upon how loud your body is shouting at you; if it is shouting loud then it is going to require a stricter level of homework and I would be in the removing camp. If you are being proactive in order to prevent disease then you are probably OK to have some grains but listen to your body as everyone is different. Reducing / cutting out carbs is a very emotive subject, especially when you start talking about removing people's daily bread, but so many people are reacting to gluten in wheat products it can be a simple way to improve health.

WHY IS GLUTEN SO BAD?
We have been eating gluten for centuries, so why now is it causing so many problems? Firstly, the gluten content in grains has increased so people can have their bouncy, fluffy loaves. Every time we eat gluten it creates micro-tears in the gut wall. If gluten were the only thing that we were exposed to that damaged the gut wall then our body would probably be able to cope, but now there are so many things, substances like Round-up, antibiotics, artificial sweeteners and food additives. These substances alter our gut bacteria and cause damage to the gut wall so the system gets overloaded and cannot keep up with the repairs. If you remember from the GUT Chapter, having a robust gut wall that does not let foreign substances through is vital for long-term good health. If we have proteins / toxins leaking through into the bloodstream this sets off the immune system, which puts the body into an inflammatory state. If we are reacting to gluten then it is likely that we may be cross-reacting to other grains as well, so if you are going to avoid gluten I would recommend cutting out all grains and see how your body reacts. Once things have improved you can always experiment with introducing some of the non-gluten grains and see if your body is happy with them.

Something I feel is very important to raise at this point is that by cutting out grains in your diet you will be cutting out a huge amount of prebiotic foods – these are the foods that feed the good bacteria. Up to 80% of our prebiotics come from grains, so if you are cutting them out it is vital that you make sure that you are replacing with lots of other prebiotics. These are:

Onions, leeks, garlic, asparagus, chicory, Jerusalem artichoke, broccoli, Brussels sprouts, cabbage, cauliflower, kale, radish, dandelion leaves, almonds, peas, pistachios, flaxseed, sweet potato.

The first reason why people improve on no grains is that they are no longer damaging their gut wall. The second is that if you remove grains then you are most likely to be dramatically decreasing the amount of carbs / sugar you are eating. In the last 5 years the prescriptions for diabetes medication have increased from 26 million to 35 million. It is a travesty that people are being given medication when they could fix themselves by simply changing their diet.

This way of eating is the basis of the paleo diet, but my version of the paleo diet includes a lot of vegetables. Our forebears would not have been tucking into woolly mammoth steak every day of the week, the majority of their diet would have been roots, vegetables, nuts and some fruit in the summer/autumn only. This way of eating does not mean that you are cutting out all carbs – there is plenty of carbohydrate content in vegetables.

GENERAL IDEAS TO HELP

Try to eat only when you are hungry – 3 meals a day is a social construct and very often we eat through habit when we really don't need fuel or feel hungry.

If you are heading for food and you are not hungry, ask yourself why, what other need are you trying to pacify with food? When emotions are too uncomfortable or painful the ego / adolescent part of our brain wants to avoid us feeling them at all costs so they get squashed down and attention is diverted to something that will distract us, be it eating, drinking alcohol, taking drugs, shopping, gambling, being overly busy etc. One of the most helpful things that my clients do is to write a food / mood diary, and I suggest that you try this for a week – it often becomes obvious if emotional needs are not being met. What those emotional needs are, is then the challenge to ascertain.

Try to eat something green with every meal. Breakfast is more of an issue but you could have a small wheatgrass shot, put some spinach in an omelette or broccoli / kale in a smoothie.

Replace carbs with vegetables – it is important to be aware of which vegetables you are eating. Many of my clients say that they eat lots of vegetables, but this entails lots of peas, carrots and sweetcorn which are some of the most sugary / starchy vegetables around. The dark green leafies are the ones to really concentrate on. We also need to be mindful that we don't include high levels of root vegetables – carrots, parsnips, sweet potatoes, potatoes. I am not saying don't have these but be mindful of how much you are having and white potatoes should definitely be eaten as a treat.

FOOD: THE LESS 'MESSED ABOUT' THE BETTER

If you don't recognise an ingredient ideally don't buy it. Most food manufacturers don't have much interest in our health and wellbeing; there are a few companies out there that are ethical and honest about what they put in their food but they are not run of the mill. Most manufacturers want to make food that tastes good, ideally with a few addictive qualities (sugar, MSG, yeast etc), and with a long shelf life to maximise profits.

This particularly includes artificially low-fat and low sugar products. Most low-sugar products have chemical sugars in to replace natural sugar, in order to keep us craving that sweet taste. With low-fat foods, firstly we need to remember that 'fat being bad for us' is untrue, but also if we remove the fat from food it doesn't taste nearly so good. The manufacturers, in a bid to keep something tasting delicious, add lots of sugar and salt. This is one of the main reasons why people on low-fat diets find it so hard to lose weight.

Buying raw ingredients is a really good way of ensuring that our food has not been messed about with. I can hear resistance already – that time factor – but cooking with raw ingredients does not have to be a lengthy process. I am inordinately lazy in the kitchen and will fling something together in 10 minutes. Chopping some vegetables up for a stir-fry or into a tray to roast, and then adding some protein to shove in the oven does not have to eat into your precious time – see recipes below for a few ideas, and there are a few recipe books in the RESOURCES section too. When we start to eat this way, we have more energy so spending a bit more time in the kitchen will not feel like such a hurdle.

EAT MORE ANTIOXIDANTS – ONE OF THE BEST WAYS TO SLOW DOWN THE AGEING PROCESS
As well as vegetables containing fibre and prebiotics (food for our good bacteria), they are also full of antioxidants, which help to combat oxidative damage in the body.

Chemistry lesson alert
Oxidation is a form of internal rusting and one of the main causes of ageing. Let me explain – all things are made of atoms and atoms have a ring of electrons around them. The electrons in the outside ring of an atom like to be in pairs, when an electron is lost this is called oxidation. The atom then becomes a free radical, which goes around trying to steal electrons off other atoms and causing a chain reaction of damage.

Main causes of oxidation are:

- Excess sugar consumption
- Stress
- Excessive exercise (I don't want to discourage anyone from going hard-core at the gym, but like with everything there is a balance to be maintained)
- Sunburn
- Eating burnt food
- Pollution and general toxic exposure
- Fighting off infections
- Chronic inflammation
- General metabolism

It is not possible to eradicate free radicals (in fact they are often used by the immune system to kill bugs) but it is a good idea to try and provide the body with a good source of antioxidants to counteract the damage they can create. Antioxidants come from brightly coloured fruits and vegetables. If you think of a pepper growing out in the sunshine, it is exposed to ultra-violet radiation just like we are, but it can't slap sunscreen on to protect itself against free radicals so it develops pigments which give it bright colour and help to counteract the oxidation caused by the sun. If you eat these pigments then you benefit from the antioxidant effect.

Eat a rainbow every day

Red foods: tomatoes, strawberries, red peppers, apples, raspberries, cherries, rhubarb, radishes, pomegranates.

Orange foods: carrots, swedes, pumpkin, sweet potato, peaches, oranges, squash, mango.

Yellow foods: marrow, yellow peppers, bananas.

Green foods: broccoli, kale, spinach, cabbage, spring greens, cucumber, salad leaves, avocado, apples, kiwi, watercress, rocket.

Purple foods: beetroot, aubergine, plums, red cabbage, blueberries, blackcurrants, prunes.

Herbs and spices with high antioxidant properties:
- Cloves
- Cinnamon – very good for helping to keep blood sugar levels even
- Oregano
- Turmeric
- Rosemary
- Peppermint
- Thyme
- Cacao
- Cumin
- Parsley
- Basil

Nutrients that are especially anti-inflammatory:
- EGCG (epigallocatechin gallate) from green tea
- Curcumin from turmeric
- Resveratrol from red wine and ginger
- Quercetin from berries, onions, kale and of course broccoli.

I have put fruit on the list above, but it needs to be kept to a minimum – the berries are the best ones to stick to, as they are the lowest in sugar.

If you have arthritis there is evidence to show that it can be helpful to avoid the deadly nightshade group of fruits and vegetables – these are tomatoes, peppers, chillis, aubergines and potatoes (sweet potatoes are OK). If you are arthritic, try cutting these foods out for a month and see if you feel any improvement.

THE VITAL IMPORTANCE OF MAGNESIUM
I don't usually advocate focusing on single specific nutrients because generally nutrients are synergistic, but in the case of magnesium I am making an exception. Magnesium is a co-factor in approximately 700 enzyme reactions in the body, vital in the production of energy, and if you are not able to produce enough energy to maintain homeostasis then the effects are wide ranging. Many of the medications we are given to deal with chronic disease deplete magnesium and in our fast-paced lives, we tend to burn through our magnesium supplies. Magnesium is our relaxing mineral – it helps to relax muscles and blood vessels which lowers blood pressure. Our soils are becoming so depleted in magnesium due to acid rain that it is hard for our bodies to replenish their supplies with diet alone. It is estimated that 70–80% of the population is magnesium deficient.

Below are some of the symptoms that indicate potential magnesium deficiency:
- Muscle cramps, twitches or tics
- Muscle weakness
- Tremors
- Thyroid issues
- Restlessness
- Anxiety and over-reaction to stress
- Hyperactivity
- Being startled easily
- Insomnia
- Osteoporosis – it is not all about calcium
- Heart arrhythmias
- High blood pressure
- Kidney stones
- Migraines

- Constipation
- Depression
- Chronic Fatigue

Top Magnesium Foods:
- Kelp
- Spinach
- Swiss chard
- Pumpkin seeds
- Dark chocolate, min. 70% cocoa solids, ideally higher
- Almonds
- Blackstrap molasses
- Brazil nuts
- Pecans
- Walnuts
- Avocado
- Dried figs

Grains have a good level of magnesium, but as I am recommending you cut down on these I have not put them on the list. Magnesium is also important for helping to digest protein and as I recommend that we have a source of protein at every meal (only a small amount) maintaining optimal magnesium levels is vital.

Supplementation with magnesium
If you are very deficient in magnesium it is difficult to replenish your supplies by just eating the above foods. Care needs to be taken when supplementing magnesium as some of the different forms are not easy for the body to absorb. The best ones to look out for are:
Magnesium Glycinate – least likely to upset the stomach – good for nerve pain

Magnesium Citrate – good for relaxing muscles

Magnesium L-Threonate – good for anxiety, depression and memory

Magnesium Taurate – good for heart issues and blood pressure

Magnesium Malate – good for increasing energy

Some people need quite high levels of magnesium initially to get their levels up so experiment with dosage; if you overdose on magnesium it is likely to give you diarrhoea but you will not have done any harm, it just means that you need to reduce your dose. Be aware that magnesium can interact with medication, so if you are taking medication please do the research to make sure that it is safe. https://reference.medscape.com/drug-interactionchecker.

LECTIN FOODS

If you are eating a healthy diet and have got your stress response under control and are not getting the results, it might be worth cutting out lectins. This is a tricky subject because many healthy plant foods contain lectins (which can be toxic to a sensitive body) and I don't want to be deterring people from eating these foods unless necessary. Lectins are proteins that plants (and animals) produce in a bid to protect themselves from being eaten by others. They are contained in all parts of the plant, the leaves, the seeds and the skins.

It has been proved that if you have a plant that is being munched by a caterpillar on one of its leaves, the lectin content of that plant will increase. When lectins are ingested by the 'predator' they can actually make holes in the gut wall leading to leaky gut, but they also manage to squeeze through these holes and get access to the whole body. Once in the body they will bind with the sugars that can be found in the cell membranes. This means that the lectins can disrupt the function of any cell by interrupting communication between them and promoting inflammation. Lectins have an important part to play in the progression of autoimmune dieases.[116] If you think this may be relevant to you read *The Plant Paradox* by Steven Gundry. Grains and legumes contain lectins, and be aware that cashews and peanuts are legumes, not nuts.

Although most plant foods contain lectins, below are the ones that contain the highest levels:

Deadly nightshade vegetables / fruit – tomatoes, aubergines, chillis, potatoes and goji berries

Pumpkins and squashes

Courgette

Cucumber – I never understood why so many of my clients have such a problem eating cucumber when they are approximately 95% water – perhaps this is why.

Melon

There are ways of reducing the lectin content of the above foods. For the fruits and vegetables, if you peel and deseed them before consuming, this will help. For the beans and legumes, pressure cooking is the most efficient way to reduce lectin content. If you don't have a pressure cooker you need to soak the beans for at least 12 hours, changing the water 3–4 times. Rinse the beans well and then bring to the boil in fresh water. Boil on a high heat for at least 20 minutes and skim off any scum, continue to boil on a lower heat for an hour or until the beans are soft.

If you are not feeling the benefits of a more paleo way of eating then keep searching; as I said before, human bodies are too sophisticated for a one-size-fits-all approach. Perhaps you need to remove all lectins; perhaps your body can't cope with histamines or oxalates in the diet or FODMAPs (Fermentable Oligo-, Di-, Mono-saccharides And Polyols – these sugars are difficult for the digestive system to break down if the digestion is not working properly and can cause symptoms) or tree nuts or eggs or soy … the list is endless – it could be purely an emotional issue. I am not going to go into the ins and outs of all of these diets as there is plenty of good information to guide you if you think any of these particular foods is a problem. However, what I will say is that very rarely are we born reacting to these foods, and in my experience unless it is a proper allergy it is possible to heal the gut, rebalance the immune system and go back to eating these foods without symptoms. Listen to your body and experiment. Yes, it can be a long process, especially when the body can sometimes cope with a food one day and another day not, bodies can have good days and bad days and their resilience levels go up and down, which can make it very difficult to work out what you might be reacting to. But stick with it – writing a food and symptom diary can really help to join up the dots. The most difficult thing is being strong willed about giving up the foods that are our favourites. Very often we crave the foods that our body is reacting to, so I would always start with cutting out these foods first.

A WORD ABOUT CALORIES

The government at the moment, in a bid to address the obesity crisis, which is costing the country approximately £45 billion a year, are concentrating on calories. They feel that it would be helpful if all foods had the calorie content put on the front of packets to make it easier. Unfortunately, they don't seem to have read the research that shows that foods with equivalent calories can have very different effects on blood sugar levels. Take a can of coke for example, which contains 26.5 gms of sugar (that is 6.5 teaspoons and 105 calories) and a large broccoli tree, which contains the same amount of calories and 3 gms of sugar. Which one is likely to fill you up more and which one is more likely to play havoc with your appetite, fat storage system and general feeling of satiety?

FAT AND CALORIES

Fatty food contains higher levels of calories (1gm of fat equals 9 calories and 1gm of sugar gives 4 calories). So, you can see why there is confusion about fat consumption making us fat, when we are adhering to the 'calories make you fat' theory. Fat does not require an insulin response in order to be metabolised in the body, so there will be less fat storage. Dr David Ludwig[117] did some interesting experiments which showed that effectively fat cells get hungry, and the more we have in our body, the more they need feeding which causes us to overeat and probably exercise less because we are feeling fatigued and lethargic.

The benefits of eating fat

Getting the body to run on fat rather than glucose means less oxidation.

Increasing fat consumption and reducing the carbs also prevents us having that post-meal energy slump or low blood sugar symptoms like feeling dizzy, irritable, shaky, lethargic.

It improves the quality of our gut bacteria – pathogenic bacteria in the gut generally like to feed on sugar, so less sugar means that they cannot thrive.

It helps brain function and brings more mental clarity because brain cells are very sensitive to levels of free radicals in the system. Burning sugar as a fuel creates more free radicals.

It helps with weight-loss – if you have taught your body to burn fat as a fuel, it can then start using up the fat stores. It is much easier for the body to extract energy from glucose and so quite understandably this is what it prefers to do. If you have been eating a carbohydrate-based diet and kept the glucose levels topped up, you will not have required your body to burn fat so you have to teach it to do this by really dropping down on your carbohydrate consumption. Statistics show that Belgium, Germany, Finland and the Netherlands, despite having the highest fat consumption in the world, do not suffer with the highest obesity rates.

It maintains healthy oxygen levels in the body. Excess glucose sticks to things in the body, including our haemoglobin, needed for transport of oxygen. Oxygen-starved cells do not have the fuel to function properly, and they can start respiring anaerobically (without oxygen); we all know the effects of anaerobic respiration if we exercise hard: it produces lactic acid (making muscles stiff and sore). A more acidic environment is preferred by cancer cells and prevents the immune system from functioning optimally.

Bad fats

These are fats that have been treated in a way that changes their molecular structure. Two of the main ways that fats have their structure altered is hydrogenation, where the oil has been bombarded with hydrogen atoms so it becomes solid and spreadable – think margarine and sunflower oil spread. The other method of damaging fat structure is by heating the fat to a high temperature; many fats have a delicate molecular structure and heating can cause this structure to change. If the body is exposed to these damaged fats at low levels it can destroy them, break them down and use the parts for other things; however, if the consumption of these fats is too high, the body gets overwhelmed and has to start using them in the structure of cell membranes. This then affects the ability of the cell to function properly.

There is much controversy about heating fats and which are the ones that are safe to heat. From my research, all fats will be damaged if you heat them to very high temperatures, so try not to frazzle your food too much. These are some fats that are more resilient than others.

- Coconut oil
- Ghee
- Butter
- Olive oil
- Sesame oil

Tips for heating / storing oils
When you are roasting any food be aware that any browned / blackened food is damaged and therefore toxic, so try not to cook them for too long, or reduce the heat of the oven. If you are frying vegetables put the vegetables in the frying pan first and then add the oil, as this protects the fat from being sizzled prior to adding the food. You can also add a little water to the pan before you add the fat – make sure that the water is not hot when you add the fat as it can cause spitting. This method lowers the temperature that the fat will reach. Fats are a really healthy food to consume, but they need to be treated with respect otherwise they become toxic. Try not to heat them too high, and ideally store them in a dark glass container in a cool place. The glass rather than plastic is to prevent hormone-disrupting chemicals from leaching into the oil and the dark-coloured glass is to prevent the oil from being exposed to too much light which can cause oxidation.

Especially good fats
Coconut oil, butter, ghee and olive oil – OK to cook with

Most nut and seeds oils (except for sunflower oil, which is higher in inflammatory Omega 6 fat) are healthy to eat, but these are for drizzling only and not cooking with.

Important reminder
If you decide to go down the increased fat consumption route, you have to really cut the carbs and the sugar.

FOOD IDEAS FOR REVERSING CHRONIC DISEASE

My intention is not for this to be a recipe book – there are millions of fabulous recipe books out there far more exciting and delicious than I could ever produce – but I have put in below some of my top recipes and ideas for helping you to change your diet for the better. Please experiment with them and add your own stamp – I generally don't like being restricted by recipes and I tend to fling things in. Sometimes the outcome of this approach is more successful than others – my family are very patient with me.

BREAKFAST

I find that breakfast is the hardest one for people to get their heads around as it is grooved into our psyche that breakfast involves lots of carbs. It requires thinking outside the box a bit – the other day I came down to my eldest son tucking into a chicken and avocado salad for breakfast.

Eggs – any which way as long as they are not with toast or dippy soldiers. You can make dippy soldiers out of paleo bread – see below for recipe.

Omelettes are a good vehicle for lots of vegetables – spinach, onions, leeks, broccoli. If you make a large frittata full of vegetables (not white potatoes) it is great to have in the fridge as an easy-to-grab snack. Or if you are really pushed for time in the morning take a slice with you but try to make sure that at some point you sit down to eat it and allow your body a bit of time to digest.

Full-fat coconut yoghurt (great levels of fat which will fill you up and keep you going) with a few spoonfuls of nuts / seeds and a large pinch of cinnamon. Cinnamon is very good for helping to balance blood sugar levels. Add some berries if you like.

As my cooking involves lots of nuts and seeds, to make it a bit cheaper I get big bags of organic nuts and seeds from http://www.healthysupplies.co.uk.

Paleo Bread
3.5oz ground flaxseed
1.5oz ground almonds
¼ cup of olive oil
⅓ cup of water
1 teaspoon of sodium bicarbonate – the Arm & Hammer brand which doesn't contain aluminium.
2 eggs
A pinch of Himalayan rock salt / sea salt
Mix all ingredients together and put into a 1lb loaf tin. Bake in a 180°C oven for 30 minutes.
You can add herbs and spices to flavor this loaf. This bread freezes well.

Alternative Granola Recipe
2oz hazelnuts crushed
2oz pecans crushed
2oz almonds crushed
2oz of sunflower seeds
2oz of flaxseed
2oz of coconut flakes
1 tablespoon of honey
1 tablespoon of molasses
¼ teaspoon of salt
Put all the dry ingredients in a big bowl together. Gently melt the honey and the molasses and add a splash of water to make it a little more liquid then you can tip it over the nut / seed mixture and mix in well. Spread out in a large baking tray and put in a 160°C oven for 15-20 minutes. Take out and allow to cool. Break up into small chunks – put in a big kilner jar or other airtight container preferably not plastic.

Grain-Free Porridge
I often quadruple the quantities in this recipe to make a big batch as it doesn't seem to last very long. I store it in a glass

kilner jar in the fridge.

¼ cup shredded unsweetened coconut

¼ cup walnuts

¼ cup sliced / ground almonds

2 tbsp pumpkin seeds / chia seeds

1 tbsp ground linseed / flaxseed

Approximately 1 cup almond / coconut / hemp milk – it depends upon how runny you like your porridge

Pinch of Himalayan rock salt

1 teaspoon honey to taste (optional – ideally not)

Depending on how fine you like your porridge you can liquidise all the nuts till fine or can leave it a bit chunky; add the almond / coconut / hemp milk and cook over a low heat for 4 minutes, then leave to stand for a couple.

Be aware that some alternative milks contain added sugar.

Smoothie Guidelines

I say guidelines as I want you to be adventurous with your smoothies; it is important that they do not have a high fruit content and also have a good dollop of protein in them.

1 portion of fruit – ideally berries as they are lower in sugar

A source of protein, either 2–3 tablespoons of nuts / seeds or nut butter (but not peanuts or cashews). The best nuts are walnuts, almonds, Brazil nuts, hazelnuts, pecans; best seeds are flax, pumpkin, sesame, sunflower, hemp, chia – experiment with which ones you like best. Or a raw egg: I know that sounds rather scary but I promise you it is not. I put a raw egg in my children's smoothies for years before they actually saw me doing it, and only then made a fuss.

Something green – spinach / broccoli / avocado

1 tablespoon of fat – coconut oil, walnut oil, olive oil etc – not sunflower

Alternative milk e.g. coconut / almond

LUNCH

If we can eat a lunch with a smaller carbohydrate content, we don't get such an insulin response which then means there is not such a post-lunch energy slump.

Salad / vegetable base – any type of lettuce, rocket, spinach, cucumber; alternatively you can have lots of raw vegetables chopped finely or chunkily depending upon your preference – see recipes for vegetable ideas.

To the base add any of the following:

A good amount of protein – fish, meat, eggs

Avocado

Nuts / seeds

Sprouted seeds

Soups are also a really good vehicle for getting vegetables in. Try lots of different varieties – I tend to roast a large tray of vegetables and then put them in the liquidiser with either some meat stock / bone broth (see GUT Chapter) or if you want it to be more creamy I use almond / coconut milk. Add salt / pepper and any herbs / spices you like. It is important that your soup meal has protein in it, so either have some of the paleo bread with it (or alternative breads, see below) or you can add nuts and seeds to the liquidiser if you like smooth soup or sprinkle them on top if you like it more crunchy. Or of course some meat / fish.

Green Bread

In a bid to help you get the green stuff in at every meal, along with lots of fibre.

1.5oz of ground flaxseed

3.5oz of ground sunflower seeds – if you like your bread more textured don't grind them

3.5oz of ground pumpkin seeds

2oz of psyllium husks

4 large eggs

2oz of sprouted broccoli seeds – you don't have to wear sandals to eat sprouted seeds and they are extremely easy to do. Try ordering a BioSnacky jar and some organic seeds for sprouting – kale and broccoli seeds are particularly good for hormone balance.

2 teaspoons of sodium bicarbonate (Arm & Hammer brand)
2 tablespoons of tamari (gluten-free soya sauce)
1 tablespoon of mixed herbs
⅓ cup of olive oil
⅓ cup of water

Mix all ingredients together and put into a 2lb loaf tin. Bake in a 200°C oven for 30 minutes.

Egg-Free Bread

Some of my clients can't eat eggs, which is frustrating for them and me, so here is a good bread with no egg in.

½ cup of ground flaxseeds
1 cup of ground sunflower seeds
½ cup of crushed hazelnuts – I use the roasted ones as it gives great flavour
1.5 cups of ground almonds
1 tbsp of chia seeds
4 tbsp of psyllium husks
1 tsp of Himalayan rock salt / sea salt
2 teaspoons of bicarbonate of soda (Arm & Hammer brand)
1 tbsp of rice malt syrup
3 tbsp of melted coconut oil
1.5 cups of hot water

Mix all dry ingredients together well in a large bowl.

Mix the hot water, syrup and oil, the hot water should melt the oil. Then add to the dry ingredients and mix well.

Place into a 2lb loaf tin that is lined with greaseproof paper and bake in a 200°C oven for 35 minutes.

Turn out and allow to cool before tucking in as it is tricky to slice when warm. This loaf freezes well. Again, you can add herbs and spices for flavour.

MY VIEWS ON MEAT EATING

In the current climate, where it is becoming less fashionable to eat meat, I find I am at odds. Human beings have always eaten meat, we are omnivores, and I see quite a number of teenagers who are struggling with deficiencies because they have become vegan. I am not an advocate of eating lots of meat and I am very aware of being grateful to the animals who have given their lives. I really hope with Brexit that we are not going to start lowering our animal welfare standards. If we were all more diligent about eating nose to tail (and not wasting food) then we would not need to be farming livestock in such great numbers. Also if we got more value out of an animal by eating all of it, then farmers could be getting a more realistic price for their livestock.

SUPPER

- Protein – meat, fish, eggs, cooked with lots of herbs or spices to add flavour.
- Vegetables – raw or cooked.
- Roasted vegetables – in my opinion I have found that most vegetables will roast with good results. These are the ones that I have tried:
- Broccoli
- Cauliflower
- Carrots
- Courgette
- Asparagus
- Aubergine
- Brussels sprouts
- Cabbage
- Fennel
- Celeriac
- Kale

- Pak choi
- Mushrooms
- Onions
- Leeks
- Garlic
- Peppers and tomatoes – technically fruit but they make good roasted vegetables
- Beetroot
- Parsnip
- Sweet potato
- Jerusalem artichoke
- Turnip
- Squash
- Mushrooms

In a bid to ring the changes with our veg – I really don't want you to get bored of them – I use different herbs and spices. You don't have to use all of the list below within each category, but hopefully it will give you some ideas.

Mediterranean roast veg – basil, oregano, rosemary, sage, thyme

Indian roast veg – coriander seeds, cumin, caraway, fennel seeds, smoked paprika, red pepper flakes

Chinese roast veg – cinnamon, cloves, star anise, peppercorns, ginger, nutmeg, licorice – or just get some Chinese five-spice. Finally, a use for five-spice – thank you Michael McIntyre for that glorious sketch.

And of course don't forget garlic, which goes with all of the above.

Things to put in a salad so it doesn't get boring:
- Rocket
- Spinach

- Celery
- Mangetout
- Chard
- Parsley
- Sprouted seeds, alfalfa or broccoli are top of my list but there are a huge number of other seeds to sprout like kale, sunflower, red clover, amaranth, cress, radish, onion, mustard.
- Green beans
- Endive
- Mustard greens
- Lettuce – not just iceberg variety
- Pak choi
- Carrot
- Beetroot
- Brussels sprouts
- Kale
- Cucumber
- Dandelion leaves – superb for the liver
- Radicchio
- Fennel
- Asparagus
- Broccoli
- Cauliflower
- Chives
- Watercress
- Tomato – just be aware that the cherry varieties, although totally delicious, are much higher in sugar.

Generally, your plate should be at least 2 / 3 vegetables. Don't stint on the fat content of the dressing. Beware of most bought dressings, they tend to be loaded with sugar. A bit of Balsamic vinegar and olive oil is quite a good option and should be sweet enough for those needing a sweeter dressing. Otherwise you can use lemon / lime juice (include the zest – important to get organic, unwaxed ones), grainy mustard with lots of olive oil or any nut / seed oils (not sunflower). Being a lazy cook, I tend to mix up a large batch and keep it in a glass bottle somewhere cool, rather than making it each time I have salad.

MORE VEGETABLE IDEAS

Put them in smoothies

Put them in omelettes or make vegetable fritters

Vegetable rice

Many of us have heard of cauliflower rice, which is just raw cauliflower whizzed in a liquidiser until it looks like rice, but you can use any type of vegetable in rice as long as you are happy with your rice not looking the right colour. Broccoli, carrots, courgette, cabbage, kale, Brussels sprouts...

Onions are not great in vegetable rice, if you liquidise them they go mushy, but you can add them finely chopped. I fry the rice in lots of olive oil and some garlic – the liquidised veg does not really need cooking, it just needs to be hot.

Sometimes I don't cook it at all and have it more like a salad, with some dressing.

SNACKS

Chocolate Bites

1 large egg

3 teaspoons of cacao powder

1 tablespoon of honey or for a slightly less sweet malty flavour

I use 1 tablespoon of rice malt syrup

Large pinch of sea salt / Himalayan rock salt

7oz of ground almonds

Beat the egg and then add the rest of the ingredients. Roll

into balls and place on a baking sheet. Cook at 180°C for 12 minutes.

Cinnamon and Honey Bites
1 large egg
1–2 tablespoons of honey – as little as you can get away with!
1.5 teaspoons of cinnamon
1 large pinch of sea salt / Himalayan rock salt
8oz of ground hazelnuts
Beat the egg and then add the rest of the ingredients. This mixture is rather sticky so won't roll into balls – I just take a teaspoon of the mixture and place on a baking sheet. Cook at 180°C for ten minutes.

Toasted Nuts
Take some raw almonds, walnuts, Brazils, pecans, hazelnuts (these are the only ones I have tried but most nuts / seeds would probably work) and spread them out on a baking tray – sprinkle on some tamari (gluten-free soya sauce) and mix the nuts around – don't be tempted to put too much tamari on or the nuts go soggy. Bake in a 220°C oven for about 5 minutes (less if it is a fan oven) then take out and mix around in the tray and put in for another 5 minutes; you are really just drying the tamari onto the nuts, not roasting the nuts too much.

Vegetable Crackers
Another use for the vegetable rice mix, and in this one you can use onions. This is a great way to get a good variety of vegetables in. These crackers are also an excellent way of using up vegetable pulp if you are juicing.
My rule of thumb is ⅔ vegetable pulp / rice to ⅓ ground flaxseed. The flaxseed helps the whole thing stick together and also ensures there is a protein and a great fibre content.
I then add tamari (gluten-free soya sauce) and usually some

mixed herbs, perhaps a pinch of chilli powder depending upon my mood.

Mix well and then spread out on a tray lined with greaseproof paper, the thickness wants to be about 1–1.5cm depending on how thick you like your crackers. If you make it thicker it will take longer to dry out. Neaten the edges and score into squares whatever size you like, I make them about 6x6cm. If you have a dehydrator put them in for 12 hours or until they are dry and crispy. If you don't have one, you can put them in a low temperature oven (about 50°C) and leave for about twelve hours (this will be less if you have a fan oven) – the temperature needs to be very low because you don't want to cook the crackers, you are just drying them out. I often turn my crackers over halfway through to speed things up.

Kale or Nettle Crisps

I firstly soak some cashew nuts overnight and whizz them – you may not need to use all of the soaking water but you want the consistency to be a thick sauce. I then add a bit of salt and pepper, possibly chilli, a smidge of honey and some tamari to taste and whizz again.

I then take the kale, remove the stalks and cut into roughly crisp-size pieces. If you are using nettles ideally pick them (with thick gloves on) in spring / early summer, so they have not got too stringy, and take off the stalks.

Tip the sauce over the leaves and mix around well – use marigold gloves for doing the nettles. Once all of the leaves have a little bit of coating then spread them out on a tray. If you have a dehydrator put them in this overnight or you can put them in a cool oven set at about 50°C and leave for about 6 hours – keep checking them. When they are totally dry and crispy they are ready.

CHOCOLATE

This is a subject very close to my heart – I adore chocolate and admit to eating it most days; however, the type of chocolate that I am having now is a far cry from the days when I could quite easily hoover down a 110g bar of milk chocolate in one sitting – never actually attempted a 200g size but I am sure it wouldn't have been a problem. I think the guilt and the shame would have got to me before my body would have said stop. Over time I have weaned myself on to a higher and higher cocoa content, so I am now very happy to munch on chocolate that is 90–100% cocoa. I also find that my capacity for consuming this type of chocolate is vastly reduced, it is so much more satisfying probably because I am not getting a sugar hit, and I also will end up feeling very wired if I have too much. Below are a couple of my recipes; feel free to play around with them, and you can use different types of nuts, but for the fruit I would stick with goji berries or cranberries as they are less sweet.

Basic chocolate recipe
8oz of cocoa butter
2oz of coconut oil
6oz of cacao powder
2 tablespoons of something sweet – I use rice malt syrup as it is low in fructose, but honey is good or even molasses if you like this flavour. I use syrups instead of grainy sugar as the latter doesn't dissolve very well so the chocolate is not so smooth. Research shows that we perceive smooth foods as tasting sweeter than grainy ones, so in a bid to trick my body into thinking it is having more sugar than it is I stick to the syrups.
Melt the cocoa butter, coconut oil and syrup gently and add the other ingredients – mix well so there are no lumps of cacao powder. Pour into a tray lined with greaseproof (approx 10"x10") and leave to set in a cool place – depending upon the time of year it may stay a bit soft out of the fridge. Cut into smallish squares; I find if it is fresh from the fridge it can

KATE CHAYTOR-NORRIS

be quite a work-out to cut it up, so you may want to allow it to come up to room temperature but once chopped up it is best kept in the fridge.

This chocolate is the base for adding all sorts of other flavours, depending upon what you like. One of my favourites is adding peppermint oil (I use doTERRA oils as they are so pure) – add 20 drops for the quantities in the above recipe.

Or you can add the zest of an organic unwaxed orange or 20 drops Essential Orange Oil (doTERRA).

Or for upmarket fruit and nut – 3oz of goji berries and 2oz of crushed nuts – my favourites are roasted hazelnuts or walnuts.

If you want a more hard-core very grown-up chocolate, don't add any syrup but you can still add the above flavours.

It was not my intention to finish my food chapter on the subject of chocolate, but from my experience it is close to so many people's hearts that I feel it cannot be ignored. It is really important that we enjoy what we are eating, and that we don't become too obsessive about cutting foods out, unless our bodies are really shouting. It is possible to train our taste buds so that we can really enjoy the healthy stuff, it just sometimes takes a bit of perseverance.

'When diet is wrong, medicine is of no use. When diet is correct, medicine is of no need'
— Ayurvedic proverb

13

A WAY FORWARD

Maintaining wellbeing is all about balance – we need to keep twiddling the dials, responding to our environment and listening to the feedback our body is giving us. It is not about wrapping the body in cotton wool, as it is good to experience a little bit of adversity. It is also important for our immune systems to be challenged and that we are exposed to oxidation to develop our innate ability to produce antioxidants … but the balance is key.

I am not aiming for perfection but I passionately believe that there is so much that we can do ourselves to heal our bodies so that we can be the best version of ourselves, rather than taking medication.

A note if you are on medication – do not stop taking it immediately: it is important that you are gentle with your body and work with it. My suggestion is that you try the ideas in this book for 3–6 months before you approach your doctor to discuss reducing / stopping your prescription. This way you will have got your body into a better place and more able to cope with the change of less or no medication. I also understand that there are people with more serious health conditions for which medication is absolutely necessary; however, that does not mean that making the changes in this book won't have a beneficial impact upon their health, after which they can then decide what medication is really necessary.

I have given you a whole mountain of information, some of it a bit depressing, and you may be feeling overwhelmed, perhaps even to the extent of concluding: 'What's the point?' I urge you not to despair. My suggestion is that you get yourself a health comrade – chose them wisely, you want to find someone who will be positive, motivating and supportive, someone who will climb down into the pit with you, and get you both clambering back up. I can't emphasise enough how beneficial it is to have someone alongside you for encouragement and to strengthen your resolve when that chocolate muffin is calling. This approach, however, is not compulsory, you may on the other hand be perfectly happy doing it on your own. If you are feeling that you need more professional guidance, ideally find a good functional medicine practitioner, who will look at the whole picture – body, mind and soul. They can guide you on your journey to optimal health.

Whichever option you go for, may I suggest that you take it slowly. I understand the people who want to achieve it all in the first 30 minutes, clear out all the rubbish food, get an allotment, plant it with cruciferous vegetables, start making kombucha, sauerkraut and kefir and sign up to yoga, pilates and mindfulness, because this is me. It is the A-type person mode of operating. If you can slow down and take things step by step, you won't wear yourself out and you will have more resolve when faced with tricky decisions. Whilst you were reading, there may have been a subject or item where you thought 'Yes that's me...' – this is a good place to start. Take that one change and work out how you can fit it into your life so that it becomes a habit – this takes discipline but I have seen it time and time again with clients. Once you have made it a habit, pick something else that resonates with you; this may seem slow but small changes can have a huge impact on your health.

There is no short-term strategy for long-term health, the

changes you make need to be for life, and once your body feels better don't be tempted to slide backwards.

If you are not getting the results, don't give up – keep searching for answers, experiment with different approaches. There will always be a solution, or maybe even several as chronic diseases usually have more than one driver.

PARADIGM SHIFT

Until core beliefs and thoughts about disease are changed we are still going to receive the message that pills can fix the problem when really it is our bodies asking us to change something, be it diet, lifestyle or unpacking some old emotional baggage that has been stored away.

The health system needs to train up doctors to practise functional medicine, looking at the whole body and recommending diet and lifestyle changes as a first port of call before prescribing medication. Doctors like Rangan Chatterjee and David Unwin are doing an incredible job, spreading the word and showing patients that they can heal themselves. There should be a functional-medicine-trained Nutritional Therapist in every GP's surgery. (I am not touting for business here, I have plenty to keep me going.)

This could put an end to so much misery, where patients are going round the houses, seeing doctors and specialists, being put on more and more medication because nothing is working. This is a tragedy; patients go to the medical profession to seek help because they believe that the medical profession knows best. I hope that after reading this book you will understand why most of the time the conventional approach doesn't help. There are some very good doctors out there who are thinking outside the box, but many of them are restricted by the current medical culture. We need more doctors who are prepared to listen to what their patients' bodies are trying to say, especially when they are expressing stress and trauma. The NHS should be offering more therapies like EMDR,

Trauma Release Exercise, EFT, yoga, meditation, breathing and mindfulness. I know that in the NHS mindfulness is now being recognised as a useful tool, but waiting lists are enormous and there are still far too many people being put on medication because it is a cheaper option.

WHAT THE GOVERNMENT SHOULD BE DOING
We need to rise up and demand that the government does two things immediately: firstly starts to subsidise healthy food and tax the manufacturers that wish to continue creating food that is making us sick. There should never be the cry 'I can't afford to eat healthily.' Secondly the government needs to stand up against Big Pharma – I know that they pay huge amounts of corporation tax and wield power, but just think how much we could save if the NHS took the proactive stance of prevention rather than squashing symptoms with medication. Our health care providers need to be presenting up-to-date and accurate information about diet, teaching stress-reducing techniques and using nutrients to work with the body and bring it back into balance.

These changes are not going to happen overnight, so in the meantime take your health into your own hands. Be brave and experiment, trust that your body knows best and will let you know when you get it right or wrong!

Number one priorities
KEEP YOUR BODY FEELING SAFE – so it can carry out all of the functions that keep it balanced and healthy.
TAKE CARE OF YOUR GUT – feed it things that will promote good bacteria – and keep the bad bacteria at bay.
REDUCE INFLAMMATION – cut down on the sugar, the most inflammatory food you can eat, and eat lots of brightly coloured fruit and vegetables. Don't rely on fruit for getting your fruit and veg intake – ideally 80% should be vegetables.

OXYGENATE THE BODY – learn to breathe properly and keep your body moving.

REDUCE EXPOSURE TO TOXINS – get savvy about what is in things and look after your liver. In particular protect yourself as much as possible against EMR and campaign against 5G in any way that you can.

ENSURE A NUTRIENT-DENSE DIET – all healthy food has medicinal qualities, so listen to what your body is really asking for: it won't be sugar! Allow the body time to digest.

If you are not getting the right answers and results please don't give up; we are complex beings and life on earth provides a challenging adventure. We have been given miraculous bodies that communicate with us. If we can only take the time to listen and understand what they are saying, so that they can operate in an energetic, pain-free and joyous way.

> To each is given a Book of Rules
> A shapeless mass and a bag of tools
> For each may carve ere life is flown
> A stumbling block or a stepping stone
>
> — R. Lee Sharpe 'Builders for Eternity'

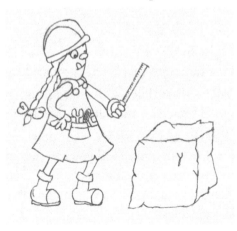

RESOURCES AND FURTHER READING

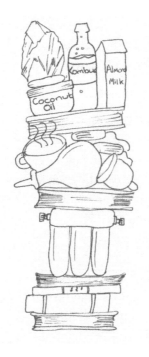

If you are looking for a registered Nutritional Therapist to work with look at the BANT website: https://bant.org.uk

BOOKS
Biology of Belief by Bruce Lipton
Daring Greatly by Brené Brown – in fact any of her books
Why Isn't My Brain Working? by Datis Kharrazian
Why Do I Still Have Thyroid Symptoms? When My Lab Tests Are

Normal by Datis Kharrazian
Grain Brain by David Perlmutter
Food Fix by Mark Hyman
Anatomy of the Spirit by Caroline Myss
The Body Keeps the Score by Bessel van der Kolk
Recovery of your Inner Child by Lucia Capacchione
Shake it Off Naturally by David Berceli
Regenerate by Sayer Ji
Human Heart, Cosmic Heart by Thomas Cowan
Spirit & Earth by Adrian Incledon-Webber and Tim Walter
The Magnesium Miracle by Carolyn Dean
Anything by Dr Rangan Chatterjee

RECIPE BOOKS
Practical Paleo by Diane Sanfilippo
The Autoimmune Paleo Cookbook by Mickey Trescott
Nom Nom Paleo by Michelle Tam and Henry Fong
The Paleo Healing Cookbook by Rachael Bryant
The Doctor's Kitchen by Rupy Aujla
Recipe books by Tom Kerridge

MEDSCAPE DRUG INTERACTION CHECKER
https://reference.medscape.com/drug-interactionchecker

WATER FILTERS
https://www.uk-water-filters.co.uk – Use reverse osmosis filter to take out all toxins including oestrogen – if you can't fit one of these in, 'Keep your own tap water' filter is the next best thing – it won't filter out oestrogen but it will filter most of the other toxic elements out.

PLASTIC-FREE WATER BOTTLES
One Green Bottle
S'well

ALTERNATIVES TO CLINGFILM
Silicon food covers – https://www.amazon.co.uk/
DigHealth-Expandable-Containers-Dishwasher-Microwave/
dp/B07DKDC1NK
Beeswax wrappers – https://www.amazon.co.uk/Bees-Bees-
wax-Sandwich-Wrappers-Washable/dp/B07MP1SQMR

BONE BROTH – *very good quality freeze dried*
https://drgusnutrition.co.uk

GROUNDING ITEMS
https://www.groundology.co.uk

TOXIN-FREE TOILETRIES
Green People
Sukin
Organic Pharmacy
Weleda
REN
Boobalou for a lot of plastic-free eco-friendly household and
personal hygiene products
Non-toxic nail varnish brands – London Grace, Little BU,
Dr's Remedy
Non-toxic self-tan – Green People or Chocolate Sun
products

SANITARYWARE
Natracare for organic tampons, pads liners and wipes
For mooncups – https://www.mooncup.co.uk

THERMOGRAPHY
https://medscans.co.uk

HAIR COLOUR
https://www.itspure.co.uk

For hair dye – if you need your hair lightening I have not found a totally chemical-free one but the best that I have found is Naturtint.

TOXIN-FREE HOUSEHOLD CLEANERS
Ecoleaf
Faith in Nature
Big Green Smile
Method

NITRATE-FREE BACON AND HAM
Finnebrogue Naked Bacon and Ham

ENVIRONMENTAL WORKING GROUP is a very useful resource for looking up ingredients to see if they are toxic.

SKIN
The Ordinary
Evolve Organic Beauty
House of Life London
Green People
Sukin

MEDITATION
Headspace app
Calm app
Ziva Meditation
Jason Stephenson

WEBSITE FOR PSYCH-K®
https://psych-k.com
Eye movement desensitisation and reprocessing – https://emdrassociation.org.uk
Trauma release exercise – https://traumaprevention.com

Emotional freedom technique – https://www.thetappingsolu-
tion.com/what-is-eft-tapping/

TOXIN-FREE HOUSEHOLD FURNISHINGS
https://drapersorganic.co.uk – hemp shower curtains
https://www.greenwoodsfurniture.co.uk/Furniture-hand-
made-in-the-UK
https://www.cottonsafenaturalmattress.co.uk/natural-mat-
tresses/pure-choice-bed-mattress/
https://www.4living.co.uk/search.php?search_query=
organic+mattresses – for organic pillows, matresses and
duvets
https://cambridgefutons.com/about-us/ – uses chemical-free
fire retardant treated fabrics
http://nutshellpaints.co.uk
http://newjoy.co.uk/blog/chemical-free-childrens-furniture
http://www.ecosofa.co.uk
https://www.greenwoodsfurniture.co.uk
https://www.naturalmat.co.uk
https://www.thehempshop.co.uk/fabrics.html

ENEMA KITS
https://www.amazon.co.uk/Specialist-Supplements-Full-
Wash-Home-enema/dp/B00F1VDDXO

FOOD
Large bags of organic ground / whole nuts and seeds and
other goodies are available from the following website:
http://www.healthysupplies.co.uk/
Paleo Granola
https://marialuciabakes.com/product/keto-macada-
mia-and-coconut-granola/
https://uk.iherb.com – has some good paleo products

FERMENTED FOODS
https://www.lovingfoods.co.uk
https://happykombucha.co.uk
http://www.loadedtable.co.uk

Glossary

Autonomic Nervous System – this is the nervous system that supplies the internal organs such as the stomach, intestine, kidneys, liver, bladder, lungs, heart, genitals, sweat and digestive glands, and blood vessels. It is divided into three parts, the sympathetic nervous system and the parasympathetic nervous system which both have opposing effects upon these organs and the enteric nervous system (see below).

Cerebrospinal Fluid – this is a clear fluid found in the brain and the spinal cord. Its function is three-fold: to cushion the brain and spinal cord from trauma, deliver nutrients to the nervous system tissue and to remove waste.

Chi or Qi – is the life force of any living being, it can be thought of as a form of bio-electromagnetic energy. It flows through the body in pathways known as meridians.

Circadian Rhythm – is a 24-hour internal body clock (also observed in plants) which mostly affects the sleep wake cycle but also eating habits, hormone release, digestion and body temperature. It can be affected by light exposure and to a lesser degree temperature.

Endocrine System – is a collection of glands that produce and secrete hormones for a wide variety of functions in the body including respiration, reproduction, sexual development, growth, metabolism, sensory perception and movement.

Endogenous – arising or originating from within the organism.

Enteric Nervous System – this is part of the autonomic system that controls the gastrointestinal tract. It controls gut movement and the control of fluid exchange between the gut and its lumen. It can operate independently of the central nervous system so has often been referred to as our second brain.

Fibrinogen – is a blood protein made in the liver. During any tissue or vascular injury it is converted by thrombin to fibrin which is used in a blood clot. Fibrinogen levels are an accurate risk factor for cardiovascular disease.

Glycemic Index (GI) – is the value applied to foods depending upon how they affect blood glucose levels. A low GI means that the carbohydrate will be converted into glucose slowly and released steadily. A high GI means that the carbohydrate will be converted into glucose quickly and there will be a fast release into the bloodstream.

Hippocampus – a major part of the limbic system in the brain. It plays an important role in the consolidation of short- and long-term memories and also spatial memory, vital for navigation.

Homeostasis – is the state of a balanced internal environment despite what the outside world is doing. Homeostasis means that e.g. blood sugar, temperature, pH, hormones etc will all be regulated to maintain balance.

HPA Axis – Hypothalamic-Pituitary-Adrenal Axis is our central stress response system. These organs are involved in the production of all the hormones involved in the stress response.

Intermittent Fasting – eating all of your food within a certain period within 24 hours, ideally 6–8 hours e.g. have a late breakfast and an early supper

Ketones – are what the liver produces for fuel when it starts to break down fat. Making the body run on ketones helps to balance blood sugar levels and promotes weight-loss.

Lymph System – is a network of vessels and organs that help to carry toxins, waste and other unwanted materials, it also helps to transport the immune system's white blood cells to fight infection.

mTOR Pathway – this is included in many biological functions, including cell metabolism, growth, proliferation of cells, cell survival and autophagy which is the self-digestion of damaged cells – vital in the body's defence against cancer.

Parasympathetic Nervous System – also known as the 'rest and digest' system. It helps the body to conserve energy by slowing the heart rate, increasing the activity of the intestines and glands and relaxing the sphincter muscles in the gut. It returns the body to a calm state after the fight / flight has been triggered.

Structured Water or Gel Phase – otherwise known as the fourth phase of water as it is the transition stage between water and ice. Structured water is H302 as opposed to H2O and it forms hexagonal sheets.

Sympathetic Nervous System – also known as the fight / flight system. It is constantly active to maintain homeostasis, but if triggered during stress will increase blood pressure, heart rate and blood sugar, and will suppress the immune system.

ACKNOWLEDGEMENTS

Firstly I would like to thank all of those family and friends who encouraged me to write this book. I would also like to thank Nor (a calm and reassuring presence in my life) who makes everything run smoothly, keeping the home fires burning and enabling me to follow my passion. She is also responsible for the wonderful illustrations in this book.

I also owe a huge debt of gratitude to all of my clients who have taught me so much and honoured me with their stories.

I would like to thank all of the people over the years who have supported and educated me, helping me to decipher what my body is trying to tell me when it decides not to play ball, and giving me insights into how my clients are operating. They are Marion Storer, Eileen Coffey, Liz Buckley, Nicola Jones, Sue Hibberd, Lisa Ellis, Jo Waterworth, Sarah Wilkinson, Pauline Fullam, Brenda Adey, Adrian Incledon-Webber, Rob White, Lulu Ferrand, John Roberts, Andrea Walker and Ali my street dance teacher who makes me laugh every Monday night.

I would also like to thank my 'witchy' friends, you all know who you are – the girls who are all doing the work to try and make sense of this challenging and wonderful life we have been given. Your support and encouragement has been phenomenal and invaluable.

I would like to thank my parents – Mum who was the one who sparked my interest in health and the human body. She was the forward-thinking one, taking me to see homeopaths back in the '70s when it was considered all very woo-woo, getting rid of all of our aluminium pans and hating cooking which gave me my love of it. To my Dad who taught me the value of nature, encouraged just mucking about outside and has always been supportive of anything that I have attempted.

I would like to thank Jim Holland whose encouragement and enthusiasm gave me huge confidence to promote this book.

I would like to thank Radio HP, without their services I would not have discovered Tandem Publishing and the wonderful Sam Carter who is completely responsible for turning my health ramblings into this book. I can't thank you enough.

ENDNOTES

1. https://www.ancient.eu/article/991/prehistoric-hunter-gatherer-societies/
2. YN Harari *Sapiens*, p45
3. Between 2003 and 2013 the annual average suicide rate was 1,900; in the year 2016 there were 5,668 suicides in Great Britain. This takes no account of the millions of people on anti-depressants and anti-psychotics that are having their life experience altered and often blunted by medication, or the 786,000 children in 2012 that were diagnosed with ADHD (attention deficit hyperactivity disorder), up from 92,000 in 1997.
4. Winston R, Chicot R. The importance of early bonding on the long-term mental health and resilience of children. London J Prim Care (Abingdon). 2016;8(1):12–14. Published 2016 Feb 24. doi:10.1080/17571472.2015.1133 012
5. Ainit Snir, Dani Nadel, Iris Groman-Yaroslavski, Yoel Melamed, Marcelo Sternberg, Ofer Bar-Yosef, Ehud Weiss The Origin of Cultivation and Proto-Weeds, Long Before Neolithic Farming Published: July 22, 2015. https://doi.org/10.1371/journal.pone.0131422
6. https://www.ancient.eu/article/991/prehistoric-hunter-gatherer-societies/
7. Leslie C. Aiello, Peter Wheeler 'The Expensive-Tisuue Hypothesis: the Brain and the Digestive System in Human and Primate Evolution'. Current Anthropology, Volume 36, Issue 2 (Apr. 1995), 199-221. https://courses.edx.org/asset-v1:WellesleyX+ANTH207x_2+2T2015+type@asset+block/Aiello95_expensivetissue_.pdf
8. http://ajcn.nutrition.org/content/early/2010/01/13/ajcn.2009.27725.abstract
9. Oster, K, Oster, J, and Ross, D 'Immune Response to Bovine Xanthine Oxidase in Atherosclerotic Patients.' American Laboratory, August, 1974, 41-47
10. https://www.heartfoundation.org.au/news/heart-disease-in-young-people
11. https://www.diabetes.org.uk/about-us/news/children-young-adults-type-2-rise
12. von Känel, Roland MD; Hepp, Urs MD; Buddeberg, Claus MD; Keel, Marius MD; Mica, Ladislav MD; Aschbacher, Kirstin BA; Schnyder, Ulrich MD 'Altered Blood Coagulation in Patients With Posttraumatic Stress Disorder' Psychosomatic Medicine: July-August 2006 – Volume 68 – Issue 4 – pp 598-604
13. Ernst E, Resch KL. Fibrinogen as a Cardiovascular Risk Factor: A Meta-Analysis and Review of the Literature. Ann Intern Med. 1993;118:956–963. doi: 10.7326/0003-4819-118-12-199306150-00008
14. Kisters K et al, 'Hypomagnesaemia, borderline hypertension and hyperlip-

idemia' Magnesium Bull, vol. 21, pp1315-1317, 1984

15. Laeremans M[1], Dons E[2], Avila-Palencia I[3], Carrasco-Turigas G[3], Orjuela JP[4], Anaya E[4], Cole-Hunter T[5], de Nazelle A[4], Nieuwenhuijsen M[3], Standaert A[6], Van Poppel M[6], De Boever P[2], Int Panis L[7]. 'Short-term effects of physical activity, air pollution and their interaction on the cardiovascular and respiratory system' 2018 May 2;117:82-90. doi: 10.1016/j.envint.2018.04.040. [Epub ahead of print]

16. JP Desborough 'The stress response to trauma and surgery' BJA: British Journal of Anaesthesia, Volume 85, Issue 1, 1 July 2000, pp 109–117

17. Sayer Ji, 'Chemo and Radiation Can Make Cancer More Malignant'. GreenMedInfo LLC, July 2012

18. Seneff S, et al, Nutrition and Alzheimer's disease: 'The detrimental role of a high carbohydrate diet', Eur J Intern Med (2011), doi:10.1016/j.ejim.2010.12.017

19. Westfall S[1], Lomis N[1,2], Kahouli I[1,2], Dia SY[1], Singh SP[3], Prakash S[4,5]. 'Microbiome, probiotics and neurodegenerative diseases: deciphering the gut brain axis' Cell Mol Life Sci. 2017 Oct;74(20):3769-3787. doi: 10.1007/s00018-017-2550-9. Epub 2017 Jun 22.

20. Beydoun MA[1], Hossain S[1], Fanelli-Kuczmarski MT[2], Beydoun HA[3], Canas JA[4], Evans MK[1], Zonderman AB 'Vitamin D Status and Intakes and Their Association with Cognitive Trajectory' in 'A Longitudinal Study of Urban Adults'. J Clin Endocrinol Metab. 2018 Feb 1. doi: 10.1210/jc.2017-02462. [Epub ahead of print]

21. P. Barberger-Gateau, C. Raffaitin, L. Letenneur, C. Berr, C. Tzourio, J. F. Dartigues and A. Alpérovitch 'Dietary patterns and risk of dementia' November 12, 2007, DOI: https://doi.org/10.1212/01.wnl.0000278116.37320.52

22. Lonneke M. L., de Lau Peter J., Koudstaal Albert, Hofman Monique, M. B. Breteler, Serum 'Cholesterol Levels and the Risk of Parkinson's Disease' *American Journal of Epidemiology*, Volume 164, Issue 10, 15 November 2006, pp 998–1002, https://doi.org/10.1093/aje/kwj283

23. Seshadri S[1], Beiser A, Selhub J, Jacques PF, Rosenberg IH, D'Agostino RB, Wilson PW, 'Plasma homocysteine as a risk factor for dementia and Alzheimer's disease' Wolf PA.N Engl J Med. 2002 Feb 14;346(7):476-83.

24. Michael J. Valenzuela, Fiona E. Matthews, Carol Brayne, Paul Ince, Glenda Halliday, Jillian J. Kril, Marshall A. Dalton, Kathryn Richardson, Gill Forster, Perminder S. Sachdev. 'Multiple Biological Pathways Link Cognitive Lifestyle to Protection from Dementia.' B*iological Psychiatry*, 2012; 71 (9): 783 DOI: 10.1016/j.biopsych.2011.07.036

25. https://www.researchgate.net/publication/47794995_Zn_Inhibits_Coronavirus_and_Arterivirus_RNA_Polymerase_Activity_In_Vitro_and_Zinc_Ionophores_Block_the_Replication_of_These_Viruses_in_Cell_Culture

26. https://www.gov.uk/drug-safety-update/isotretinoin-roaccutane-reminder-of-possible-risk-of-psychiatric-disorders

27. Jari Tiihonen, Jouko Lönnqvist, Kristian Wahlbeck, Timo Klaukka, Antti Tanskanen, Jari Haukka 'Antidepressants and the risk of suicide, attempted suicide, and overall mortality in a nationwide cohort.' Arch Gen Psychiatry. 2006 Dec ;63(12):1358-67. PMID: 17146010

28. Mitchell A, Steroids and depression BMJ 1998; 316 doi 24 January 1998 BMJ 1998;316:244

29. https://www.medicines.org.uk/emc/files/pil.1035.pdf

30. Buajordet I[1], Madsen S, Olsen H. Statins--the pattern of adverse effects with empahsis on mental reactions. Data from a national and an international database. Tidsskr Nor Laegeforen. 1997 Sep 20;117(22):3210-3.

31. Alice Laudisio [a1], Raffaele Antonelli Incalzi [a1], Antonella Gemma [a2], Silvia Giovannini [a3] Use of proton-pump inhibitors is associated with depression: a population-based study International Psychogeriatrics Volume 30, Issue 1 January 2018 pp 153-159

32. Harumi Okuyama, Peter H Langsjoen, Tomohito Hamazaki, Yoichi Ogushi, Rokuro Hama, Tetsuyuki Kobayashi & Hajime Uchino (2015) Statins stimulate atherosclerosis and heart failure: pharmacological mechanisms, Expert Review of Clinical Pharmacology, 8:2, 189-199, DOI: 10.1586/17512433.2015.1011125

33. Kausik K. Ray, MD, MPhil, FACC, FESC; Sreenivasa Rao Kondapally Seshasai, MD, MPhil; Sebhat Erqou, MD, MPhil, PhD; et al Peter Sever, PhD, FRCP, FESC; J. Wouter Jukema, MD, PhD; Ian Ford, PhD; Naveed Sattar, FRCPath June 28, 2010 'Statins and All-Cause Mortality in High-Risk Primary PreventionA Meta-analysis of 11 Randomized Controlled Trials Involving 65 229 Participants' Arch Intern Med. 2010;170(12):1024-1031. doi:10.1001/archinternmed.2010.182

34. Most Heart Attack Patients' Cholesterol Levels Did Not Indicate Cardiac Risk https://www.sciencedaily.com/releases/2009/01/090112130653.htm

35. M Obradovic, B L Zaric, M A Haidara, E R Isenovic, Link between Homocysteine and Cardiovascular disease February 2018, Volume 4, Issue 1, pp 1–9

36. Turner EH[1], Matthews AM, Linardatos E, Tell RA, Rosenthal R Selective publication of antidepressant trials and its influence on apparent efficacy. N Engl J Med. 2008 Jan 17;358(3):252-60. doi: 10.1056/NEJMsa065779.

37. http://www.greenmedinfo.com/article/nsaids-are-associated-in-creased-risk-myocardial-infarction-and-death

38. Bjarnason I[1], Scarpignato C[2], Holmgren E[3], Olszewski M[3], Rainsford KD[4], Lanas A[5]. Mechanisms of Damage to the Gastrointestinal Tract From Nonsteroidal Anti-Inflammatory Drugs. Gastroenterology. 2018 Feb;154(3):500-514. doi: 10.1053/j.gastro.2017.10.049. Epub 2017 Dec 6

39. Rana S. Bonds, Terumi Midoro-Horiuti. Estrogen effects in allergy and asthma Curr Opin Allergy Clin Immunol. 2013 Feb; 13(1): 92–99. doi: 10.1097/ACI.0b013e32835a6dd6

40. Annette M. Hormann, Frederick S. vom Saal, Susan C. Nagel, Richard W. Stahlhut, Carol L. Moyer, Mark R. Ellersieck, Wade V. Welshons, Pierre-Louis Toutain, Julia A. Taylor Holding Thermal Receipt Paper and Eating Food after Using Hand Sanitizer Results in High Serum Bioactive and Urine Total Levels of Bisphenol A (BPA)Published: October 22, 2014 https://doi.org/10.1371/journal.pone.0110509

41. Katy Backes Kozhimannil PhD, MPA, Rachel R. Hardeman MPH, Laura B. Attanasio BA, Cori Blauer-Peterson MPH, and Michelle O'Brien MD, Doula Care, Birth Outcomes, and Costs Among Medicaid Beneficiaries American Journal of Public Health (AJPH) Published Online: March 08, 2013

42. Bianchi VE[1]. Testosterone, myocardial function, and mortality. Heart Fail Rev. 2018 Jul 6. doi: 10.1007/s10741-018-9721-0. [Epub ahead of print]

43. Soterio-Pires JH[1], Hirotsu C[1], Kim LJ[1], Bittencourt L[1], Tufik S[1], Andersen MLInt J Impot Res. 2017 The interaction between erectile dysfunction complaints and depression in men: a cross-sectional study about sleep, hormones and quality of life.Mar;29(2):70-75. doi: 10.1038/ijir.2016.49. Epub 2016 Dec

44. Lin SM[1], Yang SH[1,2], Liang CC[1], Huang HK[3]. Proton pump inhibitor use and the risk of osteoporosis and fracture in stroke patients: a population-based cohort study. Osteoporos Int. 2018 Jan;29(1):153-162. doi: 10.1007/s00198-017-4262-2. Epub 2017 Oct 14.

45. Hung SC[1], Liao KF[2,3,4], Hung HC[5,6], Lin CL[7,8], Lai SW[7,9], Lee PC[10], Hung SR[11] Using proton pump inhibitors correlates with an increased risk of chronic kidney disease: a nationwide database-derived case-controlled study. Fam Pract. 2018 Mar 27;35(2):166-171. doi: 10.1093/fampra/cmx102.

46. Maes ML[1], Fixen DR[1], Linnebur SA[2]. Adverse effects of proton-pump inhibitor use in older adults: a review of the evidence. Ther Adv Drug Saf. 2017 Sep;8(9):273-297. doi: 10.1177/2042098617715381. Epub 2017 Jun 29.

47. Zhou Z[1], Zhang L[2], Ding M[1], Luo Z[1], Yuan S[3], Bansal MB[2], Gilkeson G[4], Lang R[5], Jiang W[6]. Estrogen decreases tight junction protein ZO-1 expression in human primary gut tissues._Clin Immunol. 2017 Oct;183:174-180. doi: 10.1016/j.clim.2017.08.019. Epub 2017 Sep 1.

48. Khalili H[1], Higuchi LM, Ananthakrishnan AN, Richter JM, Feskanich D, Fuchs CS, Chan AT Oral contraceptives, reproductive factors and risk of inflammatory bowel disease. Gut. 2013 Aug;62(8):1153-9. doi: 10.1136/gutjnl-2012-302362. Epub 2012 May 22.

49. Fromm D. How do non-steroidal anti-inflammatory drugs affect gastric mucosal defenses? Clin Invest Med. 1987 May;10(3):251-8.

50. Canyelles M[1], Tondo M[2], Cedó L[3,4], Farràs M[5,6], Escolà-Gil JC[7,8], Blanco-Vaca F[9,10,11]Trimethylamine N-Oxide: A Link among Diet, Gut Microbiota, Gene Regulation of Liver and Intestine Cholesterol Homeostasis and HDL Function. Int J Mol Sci. 2018 Oct 19;19(10). pii: E3228. doi: 10.3390/ijms19103228.

51. Li Q[1], Wu T[1,2,3,4], Liu R[1], Zhang M[1,2,3], Wang R[1]. Soluble Dietary Fiber Reduces Trimethylamine Metabolism via Gut Microbiota and Co-Regulates Host AMPK Pathways. Mol Nutr Food Res. 2017 Dec;61(12). doi: 10.1002/mnfr.201700473. Epub 2017 Nov 16.

52. Miller AB, Sears ME, Morgan LL, et al Risks to Health and Well-Being From Radio-Frequency Radiation Emitted by Cell Phones and Other Wireless Devices. Front Public Health. 2019;7:223. Published 2019 Aug 13. doi:10.3389/fpubh.2019.00223

53. Pritchard C, Silk A, Hansen L Are rises in Electro-Magnetic Field in the human environment, interacting with multiple environmental pollutions, the tripping point for increases in neurological deaths in the Western World? Med Hypotheses. 2019 Jun;127:76-83. doi: 10.1016/j.mehy.2019.03.018. Epub 2019 Mar 26.

54. http://www.dwi.gov.uk/consumers/advice-leaflets/fluoridemap.pdf

55. Yokel RA[1]. The toxicology of aluminum in the brain: a review.Neurotoxicology. 2000 Oct;21(5):813-28.

56. http://fluoridealert.org/studies/acute03/

57. https://www.iarc.fr/wp-content/uploads/2018/07/MonographVolume112-1.pdf

58. https://usrtk.org/monsanto-papers/state-court/
59. Whitewash: The Story of a Weed Killer, Cancer, and the Corruption of Science by Carey Gillam
60. Santford V. Overton & John J. Manura Identification Of Volatile Organic Compounds In a New Automobile http://www.sisweb.com/referenc/applnote/app-36-a.htm
61. J Guy W Johnson MA, MD, FRCS, The Toxic Effects of Gasoline Fumes. The Canadian Medical 1913
62. Irina N Krivoshto, BA, John R Richards MD, Timothy E Albertson MD MPH, PhD, Robert W Derlet, MD. The Toxicity of Diesel Exhaust: Implications for Primary Care. JABFM 10.3122/jabfm.2008.01.070139J Am Board Fam Med January-February 2008 vol. 21 no. 1 55-62
63. Knekt P[1], Järvinen R, Dich J, Hakulinen T Risk of colorectal and other gastro-intestinal cancers after exposure to nitrate, nitrite and N-nitroso compounds: a follow-up study. Mar 1999 Int J Cancer. 15;80(6):852-6.
64. Gudiño-Cabrera G[1], Ureña-Guerrero ME[1], Rivera-Cervantes MC[1], Feria-Velasco AI[1], Beas-Zárate C Excitotoxicity triggered by neonatal monosodium glutamate treatment and blood-brain barrier function. Arch Med Res. 2014 Nov;45(8):653-9. doi: 10.1016/j.arcmed.2014.11.014. Epub 2014 Nov 26[2].
65. Markey CM[1], Coombs MA, Sonnenschein C, Soto AM. Mammalian development in a changing environment: exposure to endocrine disruptors reveals the developmental plasticity of steroid-hormone target organs. Evol Dev. 2003 Jan-Feb;5(1):67-75.
66. Lang IA[1], Galloway TS, Scarlett A, Henley WE, Depledge M, Wallace RB, Melzer D. 'Association of urinary bisphenol A concentration with medical disorders and laboratory abnormalities in adults' JAMA. 2008 Sep 17;300(11):1303-10. doi: 10.1001/jama.300.11.1303. Epub 2008 Sep 16.
67. Jenny L. Carwile, MPH; Xiaoyun Ye, MS; Xiaoliu Zhou, MS; et alAntonia M. Calafat, PhD; Karin B. Michels, ScD, PhD Canned Soup Consumption and Urinary Bisphenol A: A Randomized Crossover Trial JAMA. 2011;306(20):2218-2220. doi:10.1001/jama.2011.1721
68. Fromm D. How do non-steroidal anti-inflammatory drugs affect gastric mucosal defenses? Clin Invest Med. 1987 May;10(3):251-8.
69. http://www.thelancet.com/journals/lancet/article/PIIS0140-6736(99)06065-1/fulltext
70. https://www.qcs.co.uk/root-canals-cause-cancer/
71. https://ijme.in/articles/lessons-learnt-in-japan-from-adverse-reactions-to-the-hpv-vaccine-a-medical-ethics-perspective/?galley=html
72. Cheryl Siegel Scott * and Jennifer Jinot Trichloroethylene and Cancer: Systematic and Quantitative Review of Epidemiologic Evidence for Identifying Hazards Int. J. Environ. Res. Public Health 2011, 8(11), 4238-4272; doi:10.3390/ijerph8114238
73. Flanagan RJ[1], Ruprah M, Meredith TJ, Ramsey JD. An introduction to the clinical toxicology of volatile substances. Drug Saf. 1990 Sep-Oct;5(5):359-83.
74. Zhang Y[1], Sanjose SD, Bracci PM, Morton LM, Wang R, Brennan P, Hartge P, Boffetta P, Becker N, Maynadie M, Foretova L, Cocco P, Staines A, Holford T, Holly EA, Nieters A, Benavente Y, Bernstein L, Zahm SH, Zheng T. Personal use of hair dye and the risk of certain subtypes of non-Hodgkin lymphoma Am J Epidemiol. 2008 Jun 1;167(11):1321-31. doi: 10.1093/aje/kwn058. Epub 2008

Apr 11.

75. https://www.ewg.org/research/canaries-kitchen#.Wiul7GWWFSw

76. Kumar V[1], Gill KD. Aluminium neurotoxicity: neurobehavioural and oxidative aspects. Arch Toxicol. 2009 Nov;83(11):965-78. doi: 10.1007/s00204-009-0455-6. Epub 2009 Jul 1.

77. https://behavioralandbrainfunctions.biomedcentral.com/articles/10.1186/1744-9081-5-46

78. Shui S, Wang X, Chiang JY, Zheng L. Far-infrared therapy for cardiovascular, autoimmune, and other chronic health problems: A systematic review. Exp Biol Med (Maywood). 2015;240(10):1257–1265. doi:10.1177/1535370215573391

79. Hölzel BK[1], Carmody J, Vangel M, Congleton C, Yerramsetti SM, Gard T, Lazar SW. Mindfulness practice leads to increases in regional brain gray matter density. Psychiatry Res. 2011 Jan 30;191(1):36-43. doi: 10.1016/j.pscychresns.2010.08.006. Epub 2010 Nov 10.

80. Sinha SS[1], Jain AK[2], Tyagi S[3], Gupta SK[4], Mahajan AS[2] Effect of 6 Months of Meditation on Blood Sugar, Glycosylated Hemoglobin, and Insulin Levels in Patients of Coronary Artery Disease. Int J Yoga. 2018 May-Aug;11(2):122-128. doi: 10.4103/ijoy.IJOY_30_17

81. Bostock S[1], Crosswell AD[2], Prather AA[2], Steptoe A[1] Mindfulness on-the-go: Effects of a mindfulness meditation app on work stress and well-being. J Occup Health Psychol. 2018 May 3. doi: 10.1037/ocp0000118. [Epub ahead of print]

82. Yang H[1,2,3], Wu X[2,4], Wang M[5,] The Effect of Three Different Meditation Exercises on Hypertension: A Network Meta-Analysis. Evid Based Complement Alternat Med. 2017;2017:9784271. doi: 10.1155/2017/9784271. Epub 2017 Apr 26.

83. Househam AM, Peterson CT, Mills PJ, Chopra D. The Effects of Stress and Meditation on the Immune System, Human Microbiota, and Epigenetics. Adv Mind Body Med. 2017 Fall;31(4):10-25.

84. Hatzipapas I[1], Visser MJ[2], Janse van Rensburg E Laughter therapy as an intervention to promote psychological well-being of volunteer community care workers working with HIV-affected families. SAHARA J. 2017 Dec;14(1):202-212. doi: 10.1080/17290376.2017.1402696.

85. https://www.telegraph.co.uk/news/worldnews/europe/netherlands/10314705/Sugar-is-addictive-and-the-most-dangerous-drug-of-the-times.html

86. M. V. Sauganth Paul, Mathews V. Varghese & R. Harikumaran Nair Long Term Consumption of aspartame and brain antioxidant defense status pages 135-140 Received 12 Sep 2011, Accepted 09 Jan 2012, Published online: 02 Mar 2012. https://doi.org/10.3109/01480545.2012.658403

87. Abou-Donia MB[1], El-Masry EM, Abdel-Rahman AA, McLendon RE, Schiffman SS. Splenda alters gut microflora and increases intestinal p-glycoprotein and cytochrome p-450 in male rats. J Toxicol Environ Health A. 2008;71(21):1415-29. doi: 10.1080/15287390802328630. https://www.ncbi.nlm.nih.gov/pubmed?orig_db=PubMed&cmd=Search&TransSchema=title&term=Journal+of+toxicology+and+environmental+health.+Part+A%5B-Jour%5D+AND+2008%5Bpdat%5D+AND+splenda

88. Carrez B, Qiao L, Hebbard L The Role of Fructose in metabolism and cancer Horm Mol Biol Clin Investig. 2015 May;22(2):79-89. doi: 10.1515/hm-

bci-2015-0009. https://www.ncbi.nlm.nih.gov/pubmed/25965509
89. Endocrine Society. (2014, June 23). High blood sugar causes brain changes that raise depression risk. *ScienceDaily*. Retrieved January 25, 2020 from www.sciencedaily.com/releases/2014/06/140623092011.htm
90. C Canto and J Auwerx. Caloric Restiction, Sirt1 and Longevity. Trends Endocrinol Metab. 2009 Sep; 20(7): 325–331. https://www.ncbi.nlm.nih.gov/pmc/articles/PMC3627124/
91. Meier-Ewert HK[1], Ridker PM, Rifai N, Regan MM, Price NJ, Dinges DF, Mullington JM.
Effect of sleep loss on C-reactive protein, an inflammatory marker of cardiovascular risk.
J Am Coll Cardiol. 2004 Feb 18;43(4):678-83.
92. Smith TJ[1], Wilson MA[1], Karl JP[1], Orr J[2], Smith CD[1], Cooper AD[1], Heaton KJ[1], Young AJ[3], Montain SJ[3]. Impact of sleep restriction on local immune response and skin barrier restoration with and without 'multinutrient' nutrition intervention.
J Appl Physiol (1985). 2018 Jan 1;124(1):190-200. doi: 10.1152/japplphysiol.00547.2017. Epub 2017 Sep 14.
93. Skinner MK. A new kind of inheritance. Sci Am. 2014;311(2):44–51. doi:10.1038/scientificamerican0814-44
94. Takashima Y, Guo G, Loos R, Reik W, Bertone P, Smith A, Santos F, Clarke J, Mansfield W, Oxley D, Kreuger F, Ficz G Nichols J Resetting Transcription Factor Control Circuitry toward Ground State Pluripotency in Human Volume 158, Issue 6, P1254-1269, September 11 2014
95. Mansuy I .https://academicminute.org/2014/09/isabelle-mansuy-university-of-zurich-hereditary-trauma/
96. https://medicalxpress.com/news/2013-02-life-insights-epigenetics.html#nRlv
97. https://medicalxpress.com/news/2013-01-epigenetic-reprogramming-inherited.html
98. Marta Weinstock The potential influence of maternal stress hormones on development and mental health of the offspring. Brain, Behavior, and Immunity Volume 19, Issue 4, July 2005, Pages 296-308 https://doi.org/10.1016/j.bbi.2004.09.006
99. Buss C, Davis EP, Shahbaba B, Pruessner JC, Head K, Sandman CA. Maternal Cortisol over the course of pregnancy and subsequent child amygdala and hippocampus volumes and affective problems. 19 March 2012 http://www.pnas.org/content/109/20/E1312.full.pdf
100. Abdallah B[1], Badr LK, Hawwari M. The efficacy of massage on short and long term outcomes in preterm infants. Infant Behav Dev. 2013 Dec;36(4):662-9. doi: 10.1016/j.infbeh.2013.06.009. Epub 2013 Aug 7.
101. Understanding Trauma – Integrating biological, clinical and cultural Perspectives by Laurence J, Kirmayer, Robert Lemelson, Mark Barad p.228
102. The Gifts of Imperfection by Brené Brown
103. Karen M. Grewen' and Kathleen C. Light[1] Plasma oxytocin is related to lower cardiovascular and sympathetic reactivity to stress' Biol Psychol. 2011 Jul; 87(3): 340–349. Published online 2011 Apr 29. doi: 10.1016/j.biopsycho.2011.04.003
104. Kerstin Uvnas-Moberg, E Bjorkstrand, Viveka Hillegaart, S Ahlenius,

'Oxytocin as a possible mediator of SSRI-induced antidepressant effects' Psychopharmacology 142(1):95-101 · February 1999 DOI: 10.1007/s002130050867

105. Kim, T., Shin, Y., & White-Traut, R. (2003). Multisensory intervention improves physical growth and illness rates in Korean orphaned newborn infants. Research In Nursing And Health, 26(6): 424-33.

106. Weze, C., et al (2005). Evaluation of healing by gentle touch. Public Health, 119(1): 3-10.

107. Gail Ironson, Tiffany Field, Judith Hurley, Galia Katz, Miguel Diego, Sharlene Weiss, Mary Ann Fletcher, Saul Schanberg, Cynthia Kuhn, Iris Burman 'Breast cancer patients have improved immune and neuroendocrine functions following massage therapy' Journal of Psychosomatic Research July 2004 Volume 57, Issue 1, Pages 45-52 DOI: https://doi.org/10.1016/S0022-3999(03)00500-2

108. Wood, D., Craven, R., & Whitney, J. (2005). The effect of therapeutic touch on behavioral symptoms of persons with dementia. Alternative Therapies In Health And Medicine, 11(1): 66-74.

109. Matthew J Hertenstein, Rachel Holmes, Margaret McCullough, Dacher Keltner. 'The Communication of Emotion Via Touch' Emotion 9(4):566-73 · September 2009 DOI: 10.1037/a0016108

110. Feel the Fear and Do It Anyway by Susan Jeffers

111. Loomba RS, Arora R, Shah PH, Chandrasekar S, Molnar J. Effects of music on systolic blood pressure, diastolic blood pressure, and heart rate: a meta-analysis. Indian Heart J. 2012;64(3):309–313. doi:10.1016/S0019-4832(12)60094-7

112. Doeling K, Poeppel D. Cortical entrainment to music and its modulation by expertise. PNAS first published October 26, 2015 https://doi.org/10.1073/pnas.1508431112
http://www.pnas.org/content/early/2015/10/21/1508431112

113. https://www.ncbi.nlm.nih.gov/pmc/articles/PMC3734071/

114. https://www.ncbi.nlm.nih.gov/pubmed/29470435

115. https://www.ncbi.nlm.nih.gov/pubmedhealth/PMH0012849/

116. Cordain L[1], Toohey L, Smith MJ, Hickey MS 'Modulation of immune function by dietary lectins in rheumatoid arthritis' Br J Nutr. 2000 Mar;83(3):207-17.

117. Cara B. Ebbeling, PhD; Janis F. Swain, MS, RD; Henry A. Feldman, PhD; et alWilliam W. Wong, PhD; David L. Hachey, PhD; Erica Garcia-Lago, BA; David S. Ludwig, MD, PhD Effects of Dietary Composition on Energy Expenditure During Weight-Loss Maintenance JAMA. 2012;307(24):2627-2634. doi:10.1001/jama.2012.6607 https://jamanetwork.com/journals/jama/fullarticle/1199154

INDEX